ANATOMICAL GUIDE FOR THE
ELECTROMYOGRAPHER

ANATOMICAL GUIDE FOR THE ELECTROMYOGRAPHER
The Limbs and Trunk

By

EDWARD F. DELAGI, M.D.   ALDO PEROTTO, M.D.
JOHN IAZZETTI, M.D.   DANIEL MORRISON, M.D.

Third Edition by

ALDO O. PEROTTO, M.D.

Associate Professor
Department of Rehabilitation Medicine
Albert Einstein College of Medicine
Director of Residency Training Program
New York, New York

Illustrated by
Phyllis B. Hammond
Aldo O. Perotto, M.D.
and
Hugh Thomas

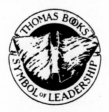

CHARLES C THOMAS • PUBLISHER
Springfield • Illinois • U.S.A.

Published and Distributed Throughout the World by

CHARLES C THOMAS • PUBLISHER
2600 South First Street
Springfield, Illinois 62794-9265

© *1994 by* CHARLES C THOMAS • PUBLISHER
ISBN 0-398-05900-4 (cloth)
ISBN 0-398-06320-6 (paper)
Library of Congress Catalog Card Number: 93-38439
First Edition 1975
Second Edition 1980
Third Edition 1994

With THOMAS BOOKS *careful attention is given to all details of manufacturing and design. It is the Publisher's desire to present books that are satisfactory as to their physical qualities and artistic possibilities and appropriate for their particular use.* THOMAS BOOKS *will be true to those laws of quality that assure a good name and good will.*

Printed in the United States of America
SC-R-3

Library of Congress Cataloging-in-Publication Data

Perotto, Aldo.
    Anatomical guide for the electromyographer : the limbs and trunk /
by Aldo O. Perotto : illustrated by Phyllis B. Hammond, Aldo O.
Perotto, and Hugh Thomas. — 3rd ed.
        p.   cm.
    Rev. ed. of : Anatomic guide for the electromyographer / by Edward
F. Delagi, Aldo Perotto. 2nd ed. c1980.
    Includes bibliographical references and index.
    ISBN 0-398-05900-4. — ISBN 0-398-06320-6 (pbk.)
    1. Electromyography.   2. Extremities (Anatomy)   3. Abdomen —
Anatomy.   I. Delagi, Edward F., 1911–   Anatomic guide for the
electromyographer.   II. Title.
    [DNLM: 1. Electromyography.   2. Extremities — anatomy & histology.
3. Back — anatomy & histology.   4. Abdomen — anatomy & histology.
5. Perineum — anatomy & histology.   B. Muscles — anatomy & histology.
WE 500 P453a   1994]
RC77.5.A5   1994
616.7'407547 — dc20
DNLM/DLC
for Library of Congress   93-38439
                                                                  CIP

To my first granddaughter
Laura Adriana

PREFACE TO THE THIRD EDITION

As with the previous revision of *The Anatomic Guide for the Electro-myographer,* the Third Edition of this book has incorporated suggestions expressed by readers of the previous edition. It also describes techniques for approaching selected muscles which were not included in previous editions. These new muscles include:

Muscles Innervated by Cranial Nerves
This section does not include a description for every muscle innervated by a cranial nerve. It describes instead the technique for selected muscles in each cranial nerve territory. The selection was based on the ease and safety of the approach to the muscle as well as traditional use of certain muscles. These muscles include those innervated by the Trigeminal; Facial; Hypoglossal; Vagus and Spinal Accessory Nerves.

Muscles of the Perineal Region
These include the rectal sphincter, the urinary external sphincter, and the transversus perineal superficialis.

Paraspinal Muscles
This group, which is divided into the cervical, thoracic, and the lumbo-sacral muscles, also includes the Quadratus Lumborum.

Muscles of the Abdominal Wall
This group includes the Rectus Abdominal and the External Oblique.

Intercostal and Diaphragm Muscles
The last additional section describes techniques to reach the intercostal and diaphragm muscles.

The reader will also find a more detailed description of electrode insertion and a commentary contrasting the approach to muscles of the limbs. *A more detailed description was deemed necessary due to the higher degree of risk inherent in approaching particular muscles of the trunk as opposed to those of the limbs.*

The technique described for the muscles in the limbs and in the trunk are the ones used by the author over 25 years experience in performing electromyography. Only one muscle is not included in this experience and that is the diaphragm. I have had no occasion to study this muscle in a systematic way. After reading Dr. P. Saadeh's technique and doing a detailed correlation of his technique in the cadaver, I came to the conclusion that the procedure is safe and sound, for which it is incorporated in this manual.

A cross-section diagram has been added to almost all individual muscles in the limbs and the trunk in order to orient the reader in placing the electrodes.

The literary sources for the Third Edition have increased, and the following sources are added to those already presented in the second edition:

BIBLIOGRAPHY
Second Edition

Gross, Charles M. (Ed.): *Gray's Anatomy of the Human Body,* 29th American ed. Lea & Febiger, Philadelphia, 1973.

Baker-Cohen, Frances: *A Study Guide and Laboratory Manual for Human Anatomy,* corrected and expanded edition, Albert Einstein College of Medicine, New York, 1971.

Haymaker, Webb, and Woodhall, Barnes: *Peripheral Nerve Injuries,* 2nd ed. Saunders, Philadelphia, 1953.

Hollinshead, Henry: *Functional Anatomy of Limbs and Back,* 2nd ed. Saunders, Philadelphia, 1960.

Sunderland, Sydney: *Nerve and Nerve Injuries.* Williams & Wilkins, Baltimore, 1968.

Crenshaw, A.H. (Ed.): *Campbell's Operative Orthopaedics,* 4th ed. Mosby, St. Louis, 1963.

Spinner, Morton: *Injuries to the Major Branches of Peripheral Nerves of the Forearm.* Saunders, Philadelphia, 1972.

Lockhart, R.D., Hamilton, G.F., and Fyfe, F.W.: *Anatomy of the Human Body.* Lippincott, Philadelphia, 1965.

Kakamo, Kenneth: The Entrapment Neuropathies. *Muscle and Nerves,* 1:264–279, July–Aug 1978.

Lampe, Ernest W.L.: Surgical anatomy of the hand. *Clinical Symposia — Ciba, 21(3):* July–Aug–Sept 1969.

Koppel, Harvey and Thompson, Walder A.L.: *Peripheral Entrapment Neuropathies.* Krieger, Huntington, 1976.

Third Edition

Anatomical Correlates of Clinical Electromyography, Second Edition
by Joseph Goodgold
Williams & Wilkins
Baltimore, London 1984

Master Class in Figure Drawing
by Robert Beverly Hale
Watson-Guptill Publications
New York 1985

Segmental Anatomy: Application to Clinical Medicine
by Marvin Wagner, M.D., M.S.
Thomas L. Lawson, M.D.
Macmillan Publishing Co., Inc.
New York, Toronto, London 1982

Myofascial Pain and Dysfunction: The Trigger Point Manual
by Janet G. Travell, M.D.
David G. Simons, M.D.
Williams & Wilkins
Baltimore 1983

The Visible Human Body
by Gunther Von Hagens, Lynn J. Romrell, Michael H. Ross, and Klaus Tiedemann
Lea & Febiger
Philadelphia, London 1991

The Head, Neck & Trunk
by Daniel P. Quiring, Ph.D.
Revised and Edited by John H. Warfel, Ph.D.
Lea & Febiger
Philadelphia 1967

Human Structure: A Companion to Anatomical Studies
by C. Roland Leeson, M.D., Ph.D.
Thomas S. Leeson, M.D., Ph.D.
W.B. Saunders Co.
Philadelphia, London, Toronto 1972

Cross-Sectional Anatomy; An Atlas for Computerized Tomography
by Robert S. Ledley, H.K. Juang, John C. Mazziotta
Williams & Wilkins
Baltimore 1977

Anatomy: A Regional Atlas of the Human Body, Second Edition
by Carmine D. Clemente
Urban & Schwarzenberg
Baltimore, Munich 1981

Needle Electromyography of the Diaphragm: A New Technique
by Peter B. Saadeh, M.D.; Christine Fitzpatrick Crisafulli, M.D.; Julian Sosner,
    M.D. and Edna Wolf, M.A.
Muscle & Nerve 16:15–20 January 1993

Laryngeal Electromyography: Technique and Application.
by R. Blair et al.
Otolaryngology Clinic of North America 1978; 11:225

Use of Hook-Wire Electrodes for Electromyography of the Intrinsic Laryngeal
    Muscles.
Minoru Hirand et al.
Journal of Speech and Hearing Research 12; 362–373, 1969

Finally, an appendix has been added to facilitate further the use and comprehension of anatomic and electromyographic knowledge. It is hoped that this new edition will help in the development of future generations of electromyographers.

ALDO O. PEROTTO

ACKNOWLEDGMENTS TO THE THIRD EDITION

The Third Edition of this book was possible due to the support and encouragement of many people:

First, due to the encouragement of many readers who found the previous two editions useful but missing important muscles of the body.

Second, due to the strong support that Dr. Edward Delagi gave to my efforts, although he decided to stay on the sidelines for the Third Edition. I would like to express my sincerest gratitude to Dr. Delagi for all that he has taught me throughout the years. In addition to myself, hundreds of other physiatrists have been able to benefit from his teaching. His understanding of electromyography and his ability to pass this knowledge on to others are extraordinary. I consider myself very fortunate to have been able to benefit from his gifts as a physician and a teacher.

I owe special thanks to my wife, Phyllis, who not only helped me with the illustrations but was a source of unwavering support and enthusiasm throughout the entire process of revising the book.

To my son, Oscar, who did a superb editorial job on the additional sections of the Third Edition.

To my secretary, Gloria Kenny, who had the patience and understanding to put up with countless changes in the drafts of this edition and in the temperament of its author.

To my friend and colleague, Dr. Harold March, who read the manuscript and made valuable corrections, a word of thanks.

Finally would like to express my gratitude to the entire Department of Rehabilitation Medicine of the Albert Einstein College of Medicine for their constant support while I was doing this work. I extend similar words to the entire resident staff, for the encouragement they give me.

A.O.P.

CONTENTS

Section I
HAND

Section II
FOREARM

Section III
ARM

Section IV
SHOULDER JOINT

Section V
SHOULDER GIRDLE

Section VI
FOOT

Section VII
LEG

Section VIII
THIGH

Section IX
PELVIS AND HIP JOINT

Section X
MUSCLES INNERVATED BY CRANIAL NERVES

Section XI
MUSCLES OF THE PERINEAL REGION

Section XII
MUSCLES OF THE PARASPINAL REGION

Section XIII
MUSCLES OF THE ABDOMINAL WALL

Section XIV
INTERCOSTAL AND DIAPHRAGM MUSCLES

ANATOMICAL GUIDE
FOR THE ELECTROMYOGRAPHER

THE LIMBS

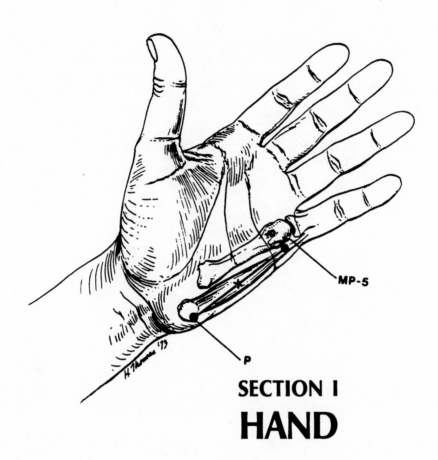

MP-5

P

SECTION I
HAND

ABDUCTOR DIGITI MINIMI

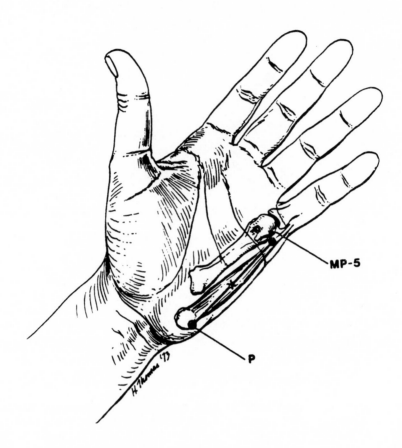

Innervation

Ulnar Nerve, Medial Cord, Anterior Division, Lower Trunk, C8, TI.

Origin

From the pisiform.

Insertion

On the medial side of the little finger into the base of the proximal phalanx.

Position

Hand in full supination.

Electrode Insertion (X)

Insert electrode to a depth of one-fourth to one-half inch at the midpoint of a line drawn between the ulnar aspects of the fifth metacarpophalangeal joint (MP-5) and the ulnar aspect of the pisiform (P).

Pitfalls

If the electrode is inserted too deeply it will be in the opponens digiti minimi.

Comment

(a) Commonly used as recording muscle for ulnar nerve motor conduction study.
(b) Involved in most ulnar nerve lesions except in Guyon tunnel entrapment when innervated through superficial palmar branch.
(c) Involved in Klumpke's palsy (avulsion of C8, TI roots).

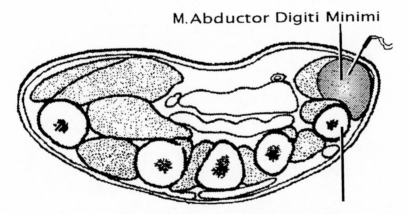

M. Abductor Digiti Minimi

5th Metacarpal Bone

Figure 1. Cross section of the hand through the junction of the proximal and medial third of the metacarpal bones.

ABDUCTOR POLLICIS BREVIS

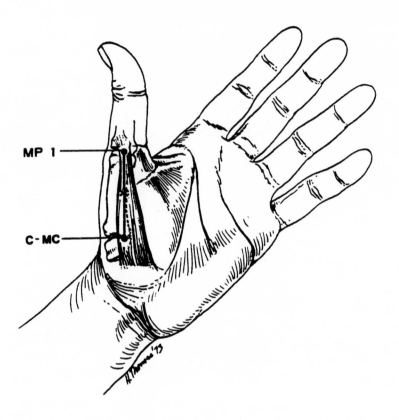

Innervation

Median Nerve, Medial Cord, Anterior Division, Lower Trunk, *C8*, TI.

Origin

From the palmar retinaculum, the tubercle of the scaphoid and that of the trapezium.

Insertion

Lateral side of the base of the proximal phalanx of the thumb.

Position

Hand in full supination.

Electrode Insertion (X)

Midpoint of a line drawn between the volar aspect of the first metacarpophalangeal joint (MP-1) and the carpometacarpal joint (C–MC). Insert to depth of one-fourth to one-half inch.

Test Maneuver

Palmar abduction of the thumb.

Pitfalls

If the electrode is inserted too deeply it will be in the opponens pollicis.

Comment

(a) Frequently used as recording muscle for median nerve motor conduction study.
(b) May be involved in all median nerve entrapment syndromes (carpal tunnel; pronator teres; ligament of Struthers) except anterior interosseus syndrome.
(c) Involved in Klumpke's palsy (avulsion of C8, TI roots).

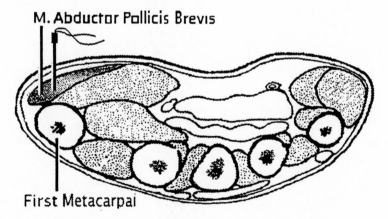

Figure 2. Cross section of the hand through the junction of the proximal and medial third of the metacarpal bones.

ADDUCTOR POLLICIS

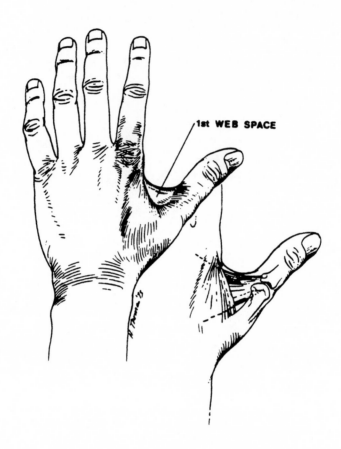

1st WEB SPACE

Innervation

Ulnar Nerve, Medial Cord, Anterior Division, Lower Trunk, C8, *TI.*

Origin

Lateral border of the third metacarpal.

Insertion

Medial side of the base of the proximal phalanx.

Position

Hand in full pronation, thumb in radial abduction.

Electrode Insertion (X)

At the free edge of the first web space. The needle is directed toward the proximal end of the first metacarpal bone.

Test Maneuver

Adduct the thumb.

Pitfalls

If the electrode is inserted too dorsally it will be in the first dorsal interosseus; if too volarly it will be in the opponens pollicis.

Comment

(a) The most distal muscle innervated by the ulnar nerve.
(b) Paresis or paralysis of this muscle results in Froment's sign (substitution of flexor pollicis longus on attempted adduction of thumb).
(c) May be involved in ulnar entrapment syndromes (Guyon's Tunnel; cubital tunnel; tardy ulnar palsy; cervical rib) and Klumpke's palsy (avulsion of C8, TI nerve roots).

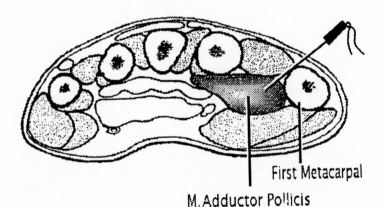

First Metacarpal

M.Adductor Pollicis

Figure 3. Cross section of the hand through the junction of the proximal and medial third of the metacarpal bones.

DORSAL INTEROSSEI

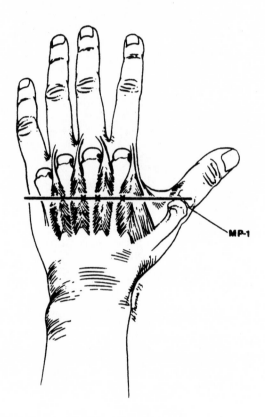

Innervation

Ulnar Nerve, Medial Cord, Anterior Division, Lower Trunk, C8, *T1.*

Origin

The first and second dorsal interossei originate on the radial aspect of the second and third metacarpal. The third and fourth dorsal interossei originate on the ulnar aspect of the third and fourth metacarpal. A small portion of the muscle originates on the opposite metacarpal.

Insertion

Base of the proximal phalanges and the dorsal digital expansions.

Electrode Insertions (X)

The common landmark for both volar and dorsal interossei is a transmetacarpal line perpendicular to the long axis of the hand at the level of the first metacarpal joint (MP–I). Insertions (Xs) are made along this line for specific interosseus muscles as indicated below:

First dorsal: Just radial to second metacarpal
Second dorsal: Just radial to third metacarpal
Third dorsal: Just ulnar to third metacarpal
Fourth dorsal: Just ulnar to fourth metacarpal

Test Maneuver

The first and second dorsal interosseus radially deviate the second and third digit, respectively. The third and fourth dorsal interosseus ulnarly deviate the third and fourth digit, respectively.

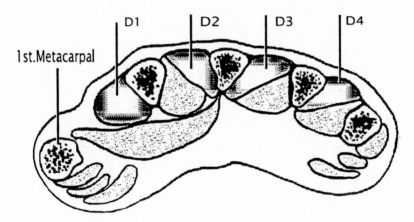

Figure 4. Cross section of the hand through the midsection of the metacarpal bones.

Pitfalls

First dorsal (DI): If the electrode is inserted too deeply it will be in the adductor pollicis.
Second dorsal (D2): If the electrode is inserted too deeply and it is angled in a radial direction it will be in the first volar interosseus; if deeper it will pierce the aponeurosis, and it will be in the adductor pollicis.
Third dorsal (D3): If the electrode is inserted too deeply and angled ulnarly it will be in the second volar interosseus.
Fourth dorsal (D4): If the electrode is inserted too deeply it will be in the third volar and if deeper, through the palmar aponeurosis in the opponens digiti minimi.

It is a common misconception that the dorsal (D) and volar (V) interosseus muscles lie in parallel planes, one completely over the other in the interosseous space, when in fact the interosseous space is divided obliquely with the greatest portion of the bulk of each muscle lying alongside the metacarpal of the digit upon which it acts; thus, orientation of the electrode along the radial-ulnar line becomes the critical factor rather than the dorsal-volar placement. (See figure page 13).

Comment

(a) There is a great variability innervation of these muscles so that they are sometimes innervated by either or both of the ulnar or median nerves.

(b) The first dorsal interosseus occasionally receives innervation from the musculocutaneous nerve (Sunderland).

(c) The first dorsal interosseus is used as the recording muscle in motor conduction studies of the deep palmar branch of the ulnar nerve. This is frequently involved in Guyon tunnel entrapment and is manifested by an increased latency of more than one ms. over that of the abductor digiti minimi on stimulation at the wrist.

(d) Frequently involved in Tardy ulnar palsy and Klumpke's palsy (avulsion of C8, TI nerve roots).

VOLAR INTEROSSEI

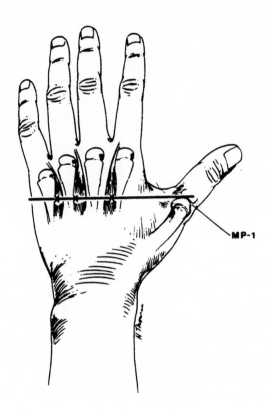

MP-1

Innervation

Ulnar Nerve, Medial, Cord, Anterior Division, Lower Trunk, C8, *TI.*

Origin

The first volar arises from the ulnar aspect of the second metacarpal; the second and third volar arise from the radial aspect of the fourth and fifth metacarpal. A small portion of the muscle originates on the opposite metacarpal.

Insertion

Bases of the proximal phalanges and the dorsal digital expansions.

Electrode Insertion (X)

Along the transmetacarpal line, insert electrodes to depth of one-fourth inch.

First volar: Just ulnar to second metacarpal.
Second volar: Just radial to fourth metacarpal.
Third volar: Just radial to the fifth metacarpal.

Test Maneuver

First volar: Ulnarly deviate the second digit.
Second volar: Radially deviate the fourth digit.
Third volar: Radially deviate the fifth digit.

Pitfalls

First volar: If electrode is inserted too superficially it will be in the second dorsal interosseus; if inserted too deeply, it will be in adductor pollicis.
Second volar: If electrode is inserted too superficially it will be in the third dorsal interosseus.
Third volar: If electrode is inserted too superficially it will be in the fourth dorsal interosseus; if inserted too deeply it will be in opponens digiti minimi.

Comment

(a) These muscles show the same variability in innervation as the dorsal interossei.
(b) Frequently involved in ulnar nerve entrapment (Guyon's tunnel; cubital canal; Tardy palsy) and Klumpke's palsy (avulsion of C8, TI roots).

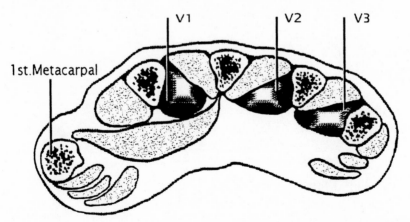

Figure 5. Cross section of the hand through the midsection of the metacarpal bones.

LUMBRICALS

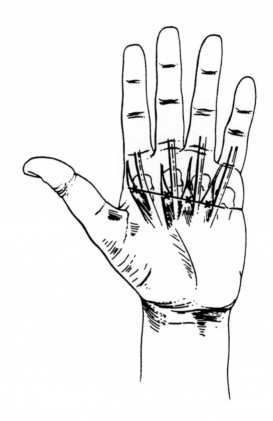

Innervation

First and Second: Median Nerve; Medial Cord, Anterior Division, Lower Trunk, *C8,* TI.
Third and Fourth: Ulnar Nerve, Medial Cord, Anterior Division, Lower Trunk, C8, *TI.*

Origin

From the radial aspect of the tendon sheath of the flexor digitoraum profundus.

Insertion

Into the radial lateral band of the dorsal digital expansion.

Position

Hand in full supination.

Electrode Insertion (X)

Just proximal to the joint and radial to the flexor tendon.

Test Maneuver

The usual method of testing lumbrical function by extending inter-phalangeal joints with the metacarpophalangeal joint in flexion is not possible because it physically interferes with the electrode. The preferred method is to maintain the metacarpophalangeal joints in extension and extend the interphalangeal joints against resistance.

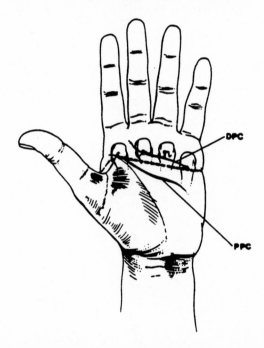

The metacarpophalangeal joints have direct relationship with both the proximal (PPC) and the distal (DPC) palmar creases. The distal crease lies over the third, fourth and fifth metacarpophalangeal joints, while the proximal lies over the second metacarpophalangeal joint. The numerical designation of a lumbrical muscle is one less than the number of the metacarpophalangeal joint it crosses, i.e. first lumbrical crosses second metacarpophalangeal joint.

Pitfalls

First Lumbrical: If the electrode is inserted too deeply it will be in the adductor pollicis; if deeper it will be in the first dorsal interosseus.

Second Lumbrical: If the electrode is inserted too deeply it will be in the most ulnar fibers of the adductor pollicis; if deeper the electrode will pierce the aponeurosis, and it will be in the second dorsal interosseus.

Third Lumbrical: If the electrode is inserted too deeply it will pierce the aponeurosis, and it will be in the second volar interosseus.

Fourth Lumbrical: If the electrode is inserted too deeply it will be in the opponens digiti minimi; if deeper the electrode will pierce the aponeurosis, and it will be in the third volar interosseus.

Comment

(a) Only 30 to 50 percent of hands have classically described innervation of first and second lumbricals being median innervated and the third and fourth being ulnar innervated.

(b) When classical innervation is present, median nerve entrapment or injury may result in involvement of the first and second lumbrical while ulnar nerve injury or entrapment may result in third and fourth lumbrical involvement.

(c) Involved in Klumpke's palsy.

FLEXOR POLLICIS BREVIS

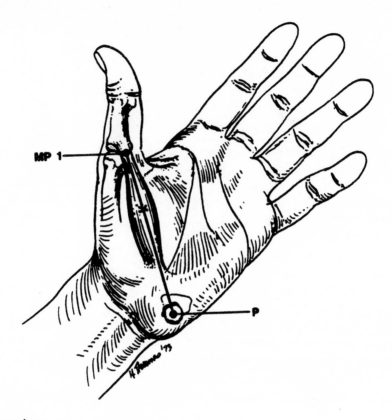

Innervation

Superficial Head: Median Nerve, Medial Cord, Anterior Division, Lower Trunk, *C8,* TI.
Deep Head: Ulnar Nerve, Medial Cord, Anterior Division, Lower Trunk, C8, *TI.*

Origin

Superficial Head: Ridge of the trapezium and the flexor retinaculum.
Deep Head: Ulnar side of first metacarpal.

Insertion

Superficial Head: Radial side of the base of the proximal phalanx of thumb.
Deep Head: Ulnar side of base of proximal phalanx of the thumb.

Position

Hand in full supination.

22

Electrode Insertion (X)

Superficial Head: A line is drawn between the ulnar aspect of the metacarpophalangeal joint (MP–I) and the pisiform (P). The needle is inserted at the junction between the middle and the radial third of this line to a depth of one-fourth to one-half inch.

Deep Head: As above but insert to depth of one-half to three-fourths inch.

Maneuver

Flex the metacarpophalangeal joint of the thumb.

Pitfalls

If the electrode is inserted too deeply it will be in the opponens pollicis, and if still deeper it will be in the adductor pollicis brevis.

Comment

(a) Two sesamoid bones are easily palpable in tendon at metacarpophalangeal joint.
(b) Due to insertion into extensor mechanism of thumb, it can extend IP joint of thumb when extensor pollicis longus is paralysed.
(c) Deep head involved in ulnar nerve injuries. Superficial head involved in median nerve injuries.
(d) Involved in Klumpke's palsy (avulsion of C8, TI roots).

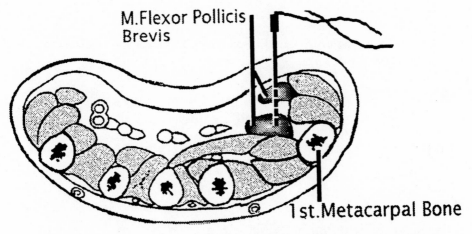

Figure 6. Cross section of the hand through the midsection of the metacarpal bones.

OPPONENS DIGITI MINIMI

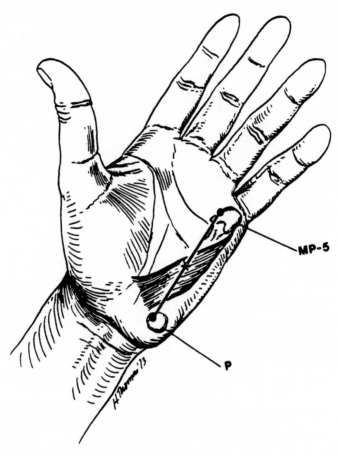

Innervation

Ulnar Nerve, Medial Cord, Anterior Division, Lower Trunk, C8, *TI.*

Origin

From the flexor retinaculum and the hook of the hamate.

Insertion

Into the medial surface of the fifth metacarpal.

Position

Hand in full supination.

Electrode Insertion (X)

Midpoint of a line drawn between the radial aspect of the fifth metacarpophalangeal joint (MP-5) and the radial aspect of the pisiform (P).

Test Maneuver

Oppose the little finger to the thumb.

Pitfalls

If the electrode is inserted too deeply it will be in fourth lumbrical; if deeper the palmar aponeurosis will be pierced, and the electrode will be in the third volar interosseus.

Comment

(a) Paralysis prevents full "cupping of hand."
(b) Involved in ulnar nerve injuries proximal to Guyon's Tunnel (cubital tunnel, Tardy palsy, Klumpke's palsy).

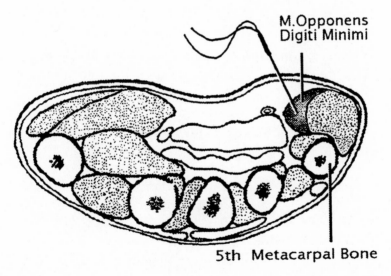

M.Opponens Digiti Minimi

5th Metacarpal Bone

Figure 7. Cross section of the hand through the junction of the proximal and medial third of the metacarpal bones.

OPPONENS POLLICIS

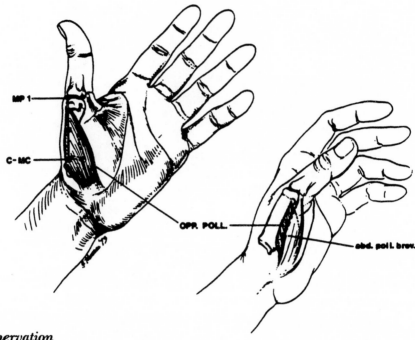

Innervation

Median Nerve, Medial Cord, Anterior Division, Lower Trunk, *C8, TI.*

Origin

From the tubercle of the trapezium and the flexor retinaculum.

Insertion

Into the lateral half of the palmar surface of the first metacarpal.

Position

Hand in full supination.

Electrode Insertion (X)

Midpoint of a line drawn between the radial aspect of the carpometacarpal (C–MC) and the metacarpophalangeal joints (MP-1). The electrode is placed between the abductor pollicis brevis and the first metacarpal to a depth of one-half to three-fourths inch.

Maneuver

Oppose thumb to little finger.

Pitfalls

If the electrode is inserted too deeply it will be in the adductor pollicis. If placed too medially it will be in the abductor pollicis brevis.

Comment

(1) The contribution to opposition made by this muscle is mainly rotation of the first metacarpal. The abductor pollicis brevis, and the adductor pollicis also contribute to the completion of this motion.

(2) May be involved in injuries or entrapment of median nerve in pronator muscle and carpal tunnel. Not involved in anterior interosseus entrapment or injury.

(3) Involved in Klumpke's palsy.

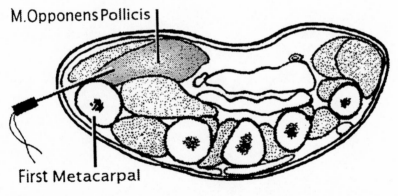

Figure 8. Cross section of the hand through the junction of the proximal and medial third of the metacarpal bones.

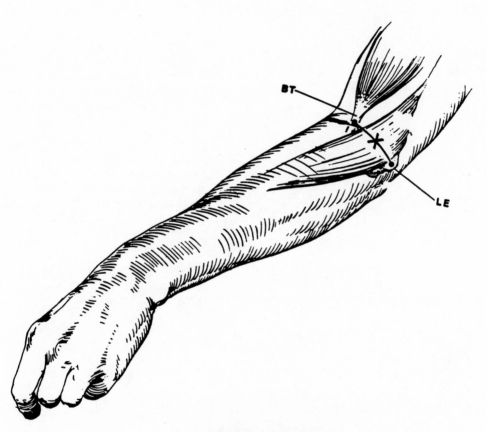

SECTION II
FOREARM

ABDUCTOR POLLICIS LONGUS

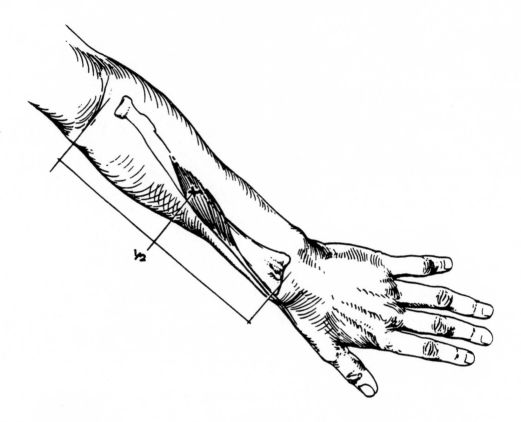

Innervation

Posterior Interosseus Nerve, Radial Nerve, Posterior Cord, Posterior Division, Middle and Lower Trunk, *C7,* C8.

Origin

From the dorsal surface of the body of the ulna, the interosseus membrane, and the middle one-third of the body of the radius.

Insertion

Lateral aspect of the base of the first metacarpal.

Position

Forearm fully pronated.

Electrode Insertion (X)

Over the shaft of the radius at mid-forearm. The electrode will travel through the extensor digitorum communis.

Test Maneuver

Radial abduction of the thumb.

Pitfalls

If the electrode is inserted too proximally it will be in the extensor carpi radialis brevis; if inserted too distally it will be in the extensor pollicis brevis; if it is inserted too ulnarly it will be in the extensor digitorum communis.

Comment

(a) Tendon involved in DeQuervain's stenosing synovitis.
(b) Involved in posterior interosseus entrapment and more proximal injuries to the radial nerve.
(c) Tendon runs through the first compartment on dorsum of the wrist.

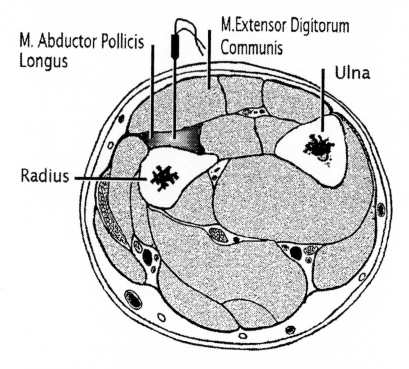

Figure 9. Cross section of the forearm through the mid-third section.

ANCONEUS

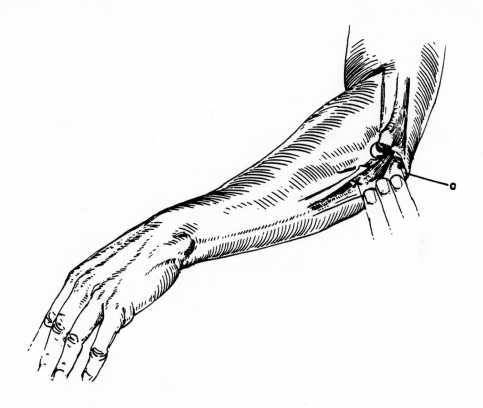

Innervation

Radial Nerve, Posterior Cord, Posterior Division, Middle and Lower Trunk, *C7*, C8.

Origin

From the posterior aspect of the lateral epicondyle of the humerus as a continuation of the medial head of the triceps.

Insertion

Lateral aspect of the olecranon process and the proximal portion of the posterior surface of the ulna.

Position

The forearm fully pronated and the elbow at ninety degrees of flexion.

Electrode Insertion (X)

Place the tip of the little finger on the olecranon (O) and ring and middle fingers along with ulna. Insert the electrode just beyond tip of middle finger, just radial to the ulna.

Test Maneuver

Extension of the elbow.

Pitfalls

If the needle is inserted too radially it will be in the extensor carpi ulnaris; if inserted too deeply it will be in the supinator.

Comment

This muscle may be considered a continuation of the medial head of the triceps to the lateral epicondyle. It is innervated by a long branch of the radial nerve, which results in its being spared except in very proximal injuries of the radial nerve.

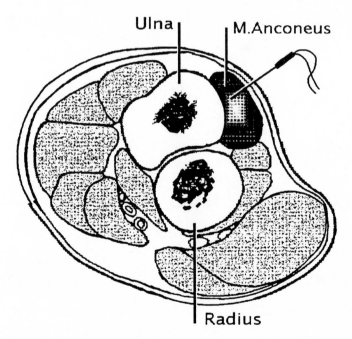

Figure 10. Cross section of the forearm through the distal elbow joint.

BRACHIORADIALIS

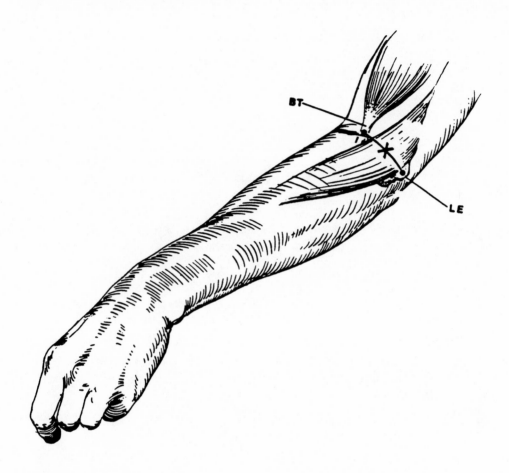

Innervation

Radial Nerve, Posterior Cord, Posterior Division, Upper Trunk C5, C6.

Origin

From the supracondylar area of the lateral aspect of the humerus.

Insertion

Lateral aspect of the radius, just above the styloid process.

Position

Forearm fully pronated.

Electrode Insertion (X)

Midway between biceps tendon (BT) and lateral epicondyle (LE) along flexor crease; insert electrode to a depth of one-half inch.

Test Maneuver

Flexion of the forearm in neutral position.

Pitfalls

If the needle is inserted too laterally it will be in the extensor carpi radialis longus.

Comment

(a) The only muscle producing flexion of the elbow supplied by radial nerve.

(b) Can act as supinator or pronator from the extremes of these positions, bringing the forearm into the neutral position.

(c) The only primary elbow flexor not supplied by the musculocutaneus nerve.

(d) Paralyzed in radial nerve injuries above or at spiral groove of humerus.

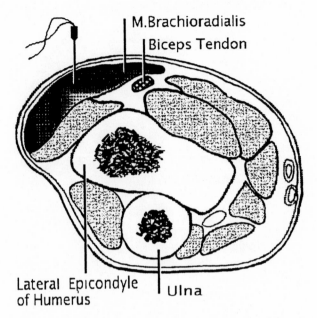

Figure 11. Cross section of the forearm through the midportion of the elbow joint.

EXTENSOR CARPI RADIALIS, LONGUS AND BREVIS*

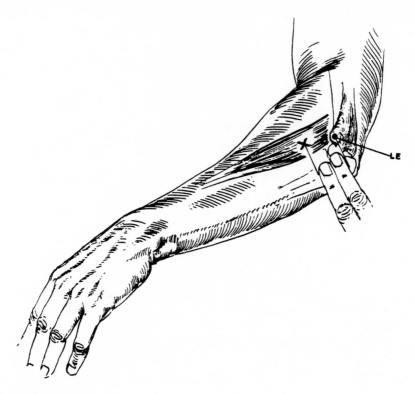

Innervation

Radial Nerve, Posterior Cord, Posterior Division, Upper and Middle Trunk, *C6, C7.*

Origin

Longus: The lower third of the supracondylar ridge of humerus.
Brevis: The lateral epicondyle of humerus.

Insertion

Longus: Dorsal surface of base of second metacarpal.
Brevis: Dorsal surface of third metacarpal.

Position

Forearm fully pronated.

---

*Because of the close anatomical and functional relationship of these muscles, the authors have found it impossible to develop a technique by which they could place the electrode in one or the other of these muscles with confidence.

38

Electrode Insertion (X)

Insert two fingerbreadths distal to lateral epicondyle (LE).

Test Maneuver

Dorsiflexion of wrist in radial deviation.

Comment

(a) The tendons of these muscles occupy the second extensor compartment on dorsum of the wrist.
(b) Usually spared in posterior interosseus syndrome but usually involved in lesions at or above the spiral groove (of humerus).
(c) Frequently involved in "Saturday night palsy."

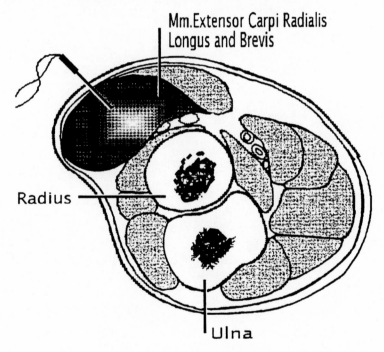

Figure 12. Cross section of the forearm through the distal elbow joint.

EXTENSOR CARPI ULNARIS

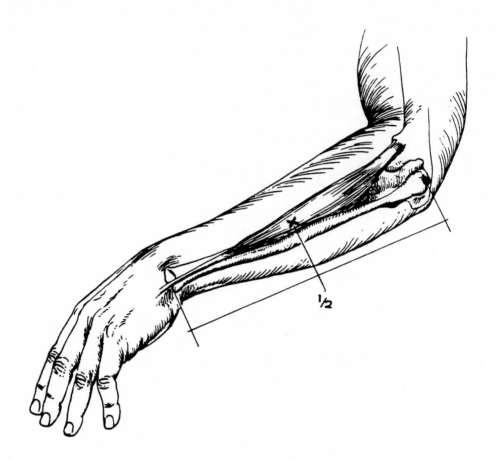

Innervation

Posterior Interosseus Nerve, Posterior Cord, Posterior Division, Upper, Middle and Lower Trunk, C6, *C7,* C8.

Origin

Lateral epicondyle of humerus.

Insertion

Dorsal surface of base of fifth metacarpal.

Position

The forearm fully pronated.

Electrode Insertion (X)

Palpate the ulna in middle of forearm and insert needle electrode just above the shaft of ulna.

Test Maneuver

Extend the wrist with ulnar deviation.

Pitfalls

If the needle electrode is inserted too radially it will be in the extensor pollicis longus, and if inserted too proximally it will be in the anconeus.

Comment

(a) The tendon of this muscle occupies the sixth extensor compartment on dorsum of wrist.
(b) Involved in posterior interosseus nerve lesions, Saturday night palsy and crutch palsy.

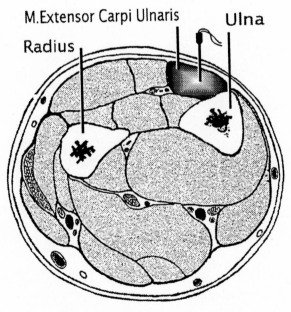

Figure 13. Cross section of the forearm through the mid-third section.

EXTENSOR DIGITORUM COMMUNIS AND EXTENSOR DIGITI MINIMI PROPRIUS*

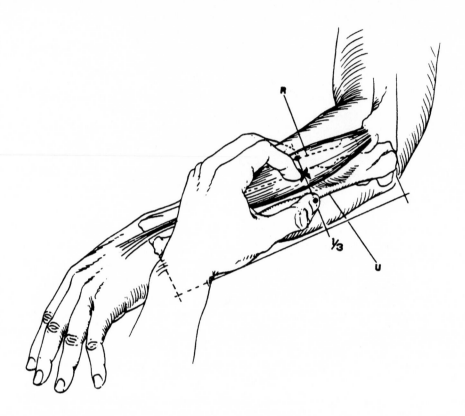

Innervation

Posterior Interosseus Nerve, Radial Nerve, Posterior Cord, Posterior Division, Middle and Lower Trunk, *C7*, C8.

Origin

Common extensor tendon from the lateral epicondyle of humerus.

Insertion

On dorsal surface of base of second to fifth phalanges of fingers.

---

*Extensor Digiti Quinti Porprius: Is most frequently a part of the extensor digitorum communis. This muscle lies very close to the extensor digitorum communis but arises from a separate slip and can be found in the mid-forearm on the ulnar border of the extensor digitorum communis.

Position

The forearm fully pronated.

Electrode Insertion (X)

Grasp the forearm at function of upper and middle third with thumb and middle finger on radius (R) and ulna (U). Then with index finger bisect these two points and insert needle electrode at tip of index finger to a depth of one-half inch.

Test Maneuver

Extend metacarpophalangeal joints.

Pitfalls

If the needle electrode is inserted too deeply it will be in the extensor pollicis longus; if inserted too medially it will be in the extensor carpi radialis brevis; if inserted too laterally it will be in the extensor carpi ulnaris.

Comment

Involved in posterior interosseus and more proximal radial nerve lesion.

(a) The tendon of the extensor digitorum communis occupies the fourth extensor compartment on the dorsum of the wrist while the tendon of the extensor digit minimi proprius goes throughout the fifth compartment.

(b) Involved in lesions of posterior interosseus nerve lesions, "Saturday night" palsy and crutch paralysis.

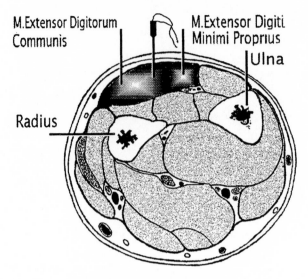

Figure 14. Cross section of the forearm through the mid-third section.

EXTENSOR INDICIS PROPRIUS

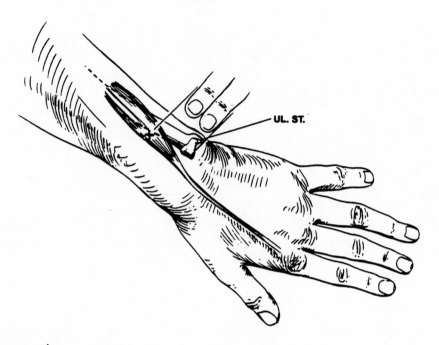

Innervation

Posterior Interosseus Nerve, Radial Nerve, Posterior Cord, Posterior Division, Middle and Lower Trunk, *C7*, C8.

Origin

Dorsal surface of lower half of ulnar shaft below the origin of the extensor pollicis longus.

Insertion

Joins ulnar side of tendon of extensor digitorum communis, which goes to index finger; terminates in extensor expansion.

Position

The forearm fully pronated.

Electrode Insertion (X)

Two fingerbreadths proximal to ulnar styloid (UL.ST.) just radial to ulnar at a depth of one-half inch.

Test Maneuver

Extend finger with flexion of other fingers.

Pitfalls

If needle electrode is inserted too radially it will be in the abductor pollicis longus; if inserted too proximally it will be in the extensor digitorum communis.

Comment

(a) Usually the most distal radial nerve innervated muscle (at times the extensor pollicis longus occupies this position).
(b) Tendon occupies the fourth compartment on dorsum of wrist with extensor digitorum communis.
(c) Used as recording muscle in radial nerve motor conduction studies.
(d) Involved in posterior interosseus and more proximal radial nerve injuries ("Saturday night" palsy and crutch palsy).

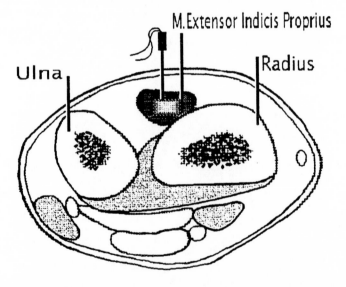

Figure 15. Cross section of the forearm through the distal third.

EXTENSOR POLLICIS BREVIS

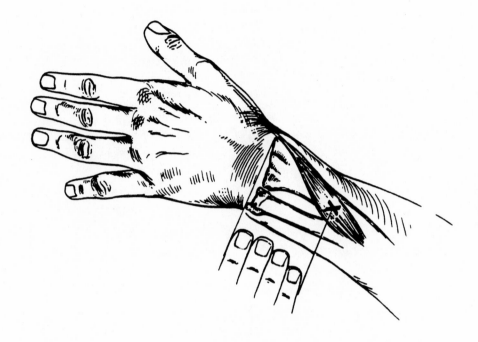

Innervation

Posterior Interosseus, Radial Nerve, Posterior Cord, Posterior Division, Middle and Lower Trunk, *C7,* C8.

Origin

Dorsal surface of radial shaft below abductor pollicis longus.

Insertion

The dorsal aspect of the first phalanx of thumb.

Position

The forearm fully pronated.

Electrode Insertion (X)

Insert needle electrode directly over the ulnar side of radius, four fingerbreadths proximal to wrist. The electrode will travel through the extensor digitorum communis.

Test Maneuver

Extend proximal phalanx of thumb.

Pitfalls

If the needle electrode is inserted too proximally it will be in the abductor pollicis longus.

Comment

(a) Tendon runs through the first compartment on dorsum of wrist. Distal to this compartment, the tendon forms the radial border of the anatomical "Snuffbox."

(b) Most distal muscle innervated by radial nerve through posterior interosseus branch.

(c) Involved in lesions of posterior interosseus and more proximal radial nerve lesions.

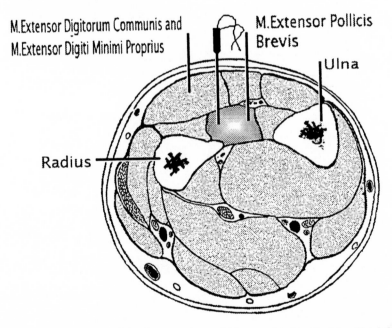

Figure 16. Cross section of the forearm through the proximal end of the distal third.

EXTENSOR POLLICIS LONGUS

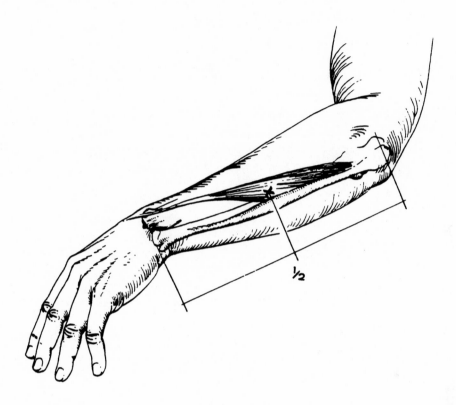

½

Innervation

Posterior Interosseus Nerve, Radial Nerve, Posterior Cord, Posterior Division, Middle and Lower Trunk, *C7*, C8.

Origin

The dorsal surface of the middle third of ulnar shaft below the abductor pollicis longus.

Insertion

The dorsal aspect of base of terminal phalanx of thumb.

Position

The forearm fully pronated.

Electrode Insertion (X)

At mid-forearm insert needle electrode along radial border of ulnar. The electrode will travel through the extensor carpa ulnaris.

Test Maneuver

Extend distal phalanx of thumb.

Pitfalls

If the needle electrode is inserted too ulnarly it will be in the extensor digitorum communis; if inserted too proximally it will be in the abductor pollicis longus.

Comment

(1) Involved in posterior interosseus and more proximal radial nerve lesions.
(2) When paralyzed, the flexor pollicis brevis may extend terminal phalanx weakly and give false impression of intact extensor pollicis longus.
(3) The tendon of this muscle occupies the third extensor compartment on the dorsum of the wrist. Distal to this compartment the tendon forms the ulnar border of the "Snuffbox."

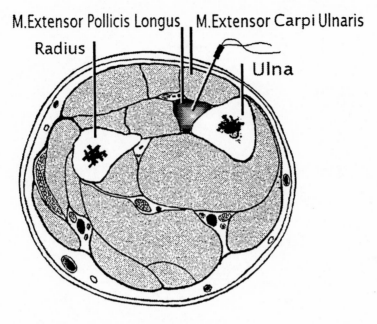

M.Extensor Pollicis Longus   M.Extensor Carpi Ulnaris

Radius

Ulna

Figure 17. Cross section of the forearm through the distal middle third.

FLEXOR CARPI RADIALIS

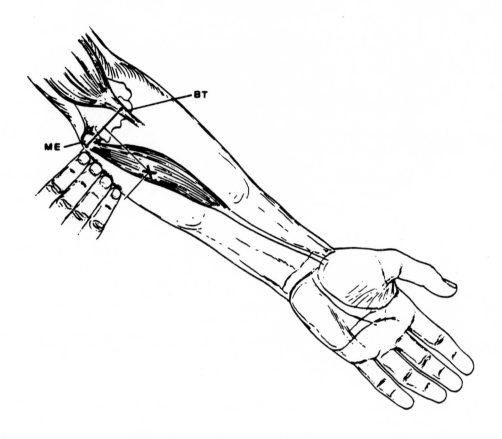

Innervation

Median Nerve, Lateral and Medial Cord, Anterior, Divisions, Upper, Middle and Lower Trunk, C6, *C7*, C8.

Origin

Common tendon from medial epicondyle of humerus.

Insertion

Volar surface of base of second metacarpal.

Position

The forearm fully supinated.

Electrode Insertion (X)

Three to four fingerbreadths distal to the midpoint of a line connecting the medial epicondyle (ME) and biceps tendon (BT).

Test Maneuver

Flexion of wrist with radial deviation.

Pitfalls

If the needle electrode is inserted too deeply it will be in the flexor digitorum sublimus; if deeper it will be in the flexor pollicis longus. If inserted too laterally it will be in the pronator teres, and if inserted too medially it will be in the palmaris longus.

Comment

(a) The median nerve runs just ulnar to its tendon as it crosses the volar aspect of the wrist.

(b) Together with the flexor pollicis longus and the radial artery they form the "Radial Trio."

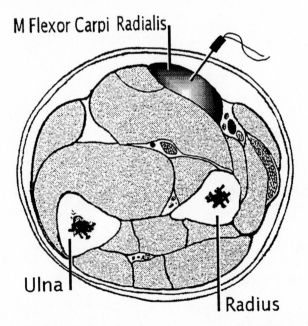

Figure 18. Cross section of the forearm through the middle third.

FLEXOR CARPI ULNARIS

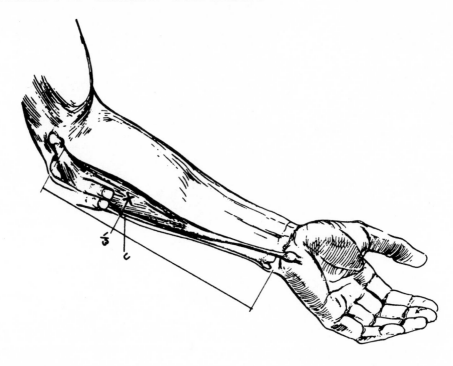

Innervation

Ulnar Nerve, Medial Cord, Anterior Division, Lower Trunk, *C8*, TI.

Origin

Common tendon from medial epicondyle of humerus, medial margin of olecranon, coronoid process, and upper two-thirds of the dorsal border of ulna.

Insertion

Volar surface of pisiform, hamate and fifth metacarpal.

Position

The forearm fully supinated.

Electrode Insertion (X)

Two fingerbreadths volar to ulna (U) at the junction of the upper and middle thirds of the forearm.

Test Maneuver

Flexion of the wrist with ulnar deviation.

Pitfalls

If the needle electrode is inserted too deeply it will be in the flexor digitorum profundus.

Comment

(a) The ulnar nerve is located just radial to its tendon at the wrist.
(b) Involved in lesions of ulnar nerve at or above ulnar groove.
(c) Together with the ulnar nerve and the ulnar artery they form the "ulnar trio."

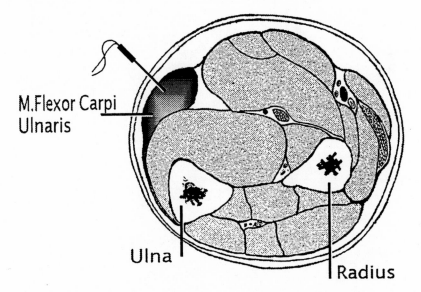

M.Flexor Carpi Ulnaris

Ulna

Radius

Figure 19. Cross section of the forearm through the middle third.

FLEXOR DIGITORUM PROFUNDUS

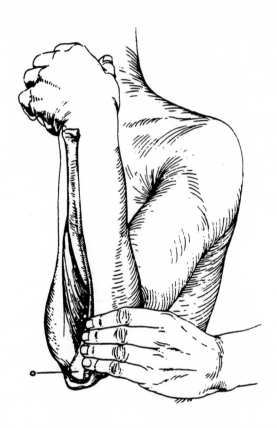

Innervation

Digits Two and Three: Anterior Interosseus Nerve, Median Nerve, Medial Cord, Anterior Division, Middle and Lower Trunk, C7, *C8.*
Digits Four and Five: Ulnar Nerve, Medial Cord, Anterior Division, Lower Trunk, *C8,* TI.

Origin

Upper three-fourths of volar and medial surfaces of ulna.

Insertion

Volar surfaces of bases of distal phalanges of four digits.

Position

The forearm fully supinated.

56

Electrode Insertion (X)

Place tip of little finger on olecranon (O) and ring, middle and index fingers along shaft of ulna. Insert needle electrode just beyond tip of index finger just ulnarly to shaft. The ulnar innervated portion is the more superficial (1–2 cm), while the median innervated portion is deeper (3–5 cm).

Test Maneuver

Flexion of distal phalanges of digits.

Pitfalls

If the needle electrode is inserted too volarly it will be in the flexor carpi ulnaris.

Comment

(a) The four tendons run across the wrist resting on the pronator quadratus. They are deep to the flexor sublimis tendon and the median nerve.

(b) The two median innervated heads are involved in anterior interosseus nerve, pronator and ligament of Struther entrapments manifested by weakness or inability to flex the terminal phalanges of second and third digits.

(c) The two ulnar innervated heads are involved in cubital tunnel entrapment and higher ulnar, medial cord and C8, TI lesions. This is manifested by weakness or mobility to flex the fourth and fifth terminal phalanges.

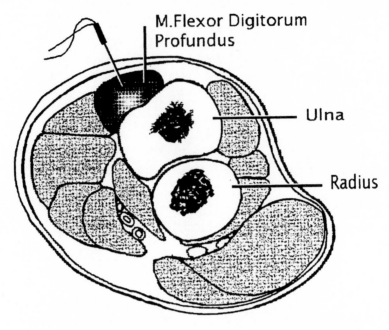

M.Flexor Digitorum Profundus

Ulna

Radius

Figure 20. Cross section of the forearm through the middle third.

FLEXOR DIGITORUM SUPERFICIALIS

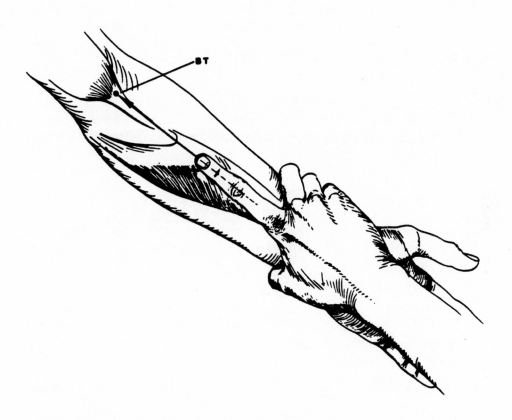

Innervation

Median Nerve, Lateral and Medial Cord, Anterior Division, Middle and *Lower Trunk, C7, C8,* TI.

Origin

Common tendon from medial epicondyle of humerus; coronoid process of ulna and oblique line of radius.

Insertion

Volar surfaces of bases of second phalanges of digits.

Position

The forearm fully supinated.

Electrode Insertion (X)

Grasp with operator's palm to volar surface of subject's wrist. Point index finger to biceps tendon (BT) and insert needle electrode just ulnarly to tip of index finger. The electrode will travel through the palmaris longus.

Test Maneuver

With the distal interphalangeal joints of three digits maintained in hyper extension, the patient is asked to flex the proximal interphalangeal joint of the free finger.

Pitfalls

If the needle electrode is inserted too radially it will be in the flexor carpi radialis; if inserted too ulnarly it will be in the flexor digitorum profundus; if too distally it will be in the tendon of the flexor carpi radialis longus.

Comment

(a) The four tendons run across the wrist in pairs: the tendons for the middle and ring fingers are the most superficial; those to the ring and little finger are deeper resting on the flexor digitorum profundus tendons. The medial nerve lies radial to these tendons as it enters the carpal tunnel.

(b) Involved in median nerve entrapments (pronator teres; ligament of Struther) and higher median nerve lesions.

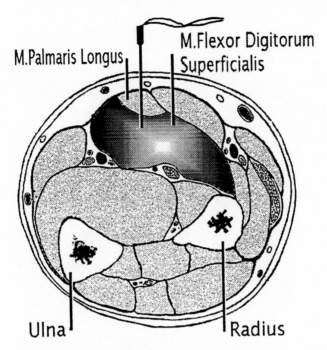

Figure 21. Cross section of the forearm through the middle third.

FLEXOR POLLICIS LONGUS

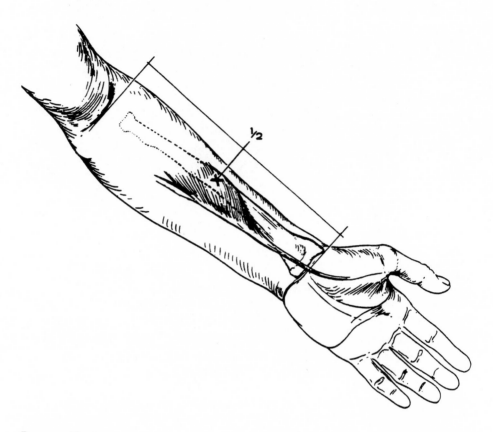

Innervation

Anterior Interosseus Nerve, Median Nerve, Lateral and Medial Cords, Anterior Divisions, Middle and Lower Trunks, C7, *C8*, TI.

Origin

The volar surface of the body of the radius from the bicipital tuberosity to the attachment of the pronator quadratus and interosseus membrane.

Insertion

Volar surface of base of distal phalanx of thumb.

Position

The forearm fully supinated.

Electrode Insertion (X)

In the middle of the forearm the needle electrode is inserted from the radial aspect just volar to the radius. The electrode will travel through the flexor carpi radialis and the flexor digitorum superficialis.

Test Maneuver

Flexion of the distal phalanx of thumb.

Pitfalls

If the needle electrode is inserted too superficially it will be in the flexor digitorum sublimis.

Comment

(a) The tendon of this muscle runs deep across the wrist, radial to the flexor digitorum profundus. With the flexor carpi radialis tendon and the radial artery, it forms the "Radial Trio."

(b) In patients with ulnar nerve lesions with paralysis of adductor pollicis, the flexor pollicis longus is substituted, producing flexion of the terminal phalanx of the thumb (Froment's "signe de journal").

(c) Involved in anterior interosseus, pronator teres and ligament of Struther entrapments.

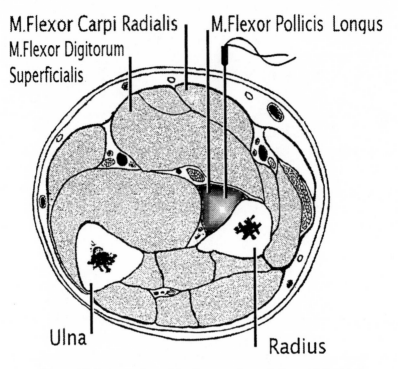

Figure 22. Cross section of the forearm through the middle third.

PALMARIS LONGUS

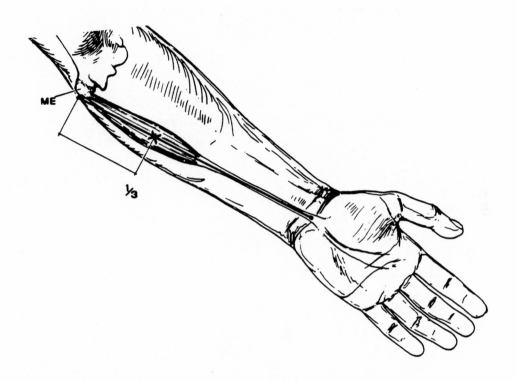

Innervation

Median Nerve, Lateral and Medial Cord, Anterior Division, Middle and *Lower* Cord, C7, *C8,* TI.

Origin

The medial epicondyle of humerus.

Insertion

The palmar aponeurosis.

Position

The forearm fully supinated.

Electrode Insertion (X)

At the junction of the upper and middle thirds of a line joining the medial epicondyle (ME) and middle of volar surface of wrist.

Test Maneuver

Cup palm of hand.

Pitfalls

If the needle electrode is inserted too medially it will be in the flexor carpi ulnaris; if inserted too radially it will be in the flexor carpi radialis, and if inserted too deeply it will be in the flexor digitorum sublimus.

Comment

(a) Absent in 10 to 15 percent of individuals.
(b) Only flexor tendon superficial to the volar carpal ligament.
(c) Involved in median nerve entrapment syndromes (pronator teres, ligament of Struther).

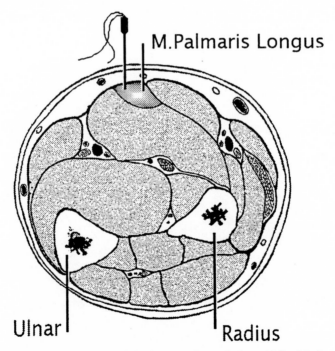

Figure 23. Cross section of the forearm through the middle third.

PRONATOR QUADRATUS

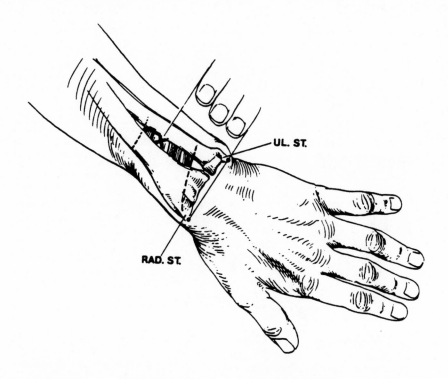

Innervations

Anterior Interosseus Nerve, Median Nerve, Lateral and Medial cords, Anterior Divisions, Middle and Lower Trunks, C7, *C8*, TI.

Origin

Lower fourth of volar surface of ulna.

Insertion

Lower fourth of lateral border and volar surface of shaft of radius.

Position

The forearm fully pronated.

Electrode Insertion (X)

Three fingerbreadths proximal to midpoint of a line connecting the radial (RAD.ST.) and ulnar styloids (UL.ST.); insert needle electrode through the interosseus membrane to a depth of approximately three-quarter inches.

Test Maneuver

Pronation of forearm.

Pitfalls

If the needle electrode is inserted too deeply, it will be in the flexor digitorum sublimis.

Comment

(a) The most distal muscle innervated by the anterior interosseus nerve.

(b) Involved in median nerve entrapment syndromes (anterior interosseus, pronator teres; ligament of Struther).

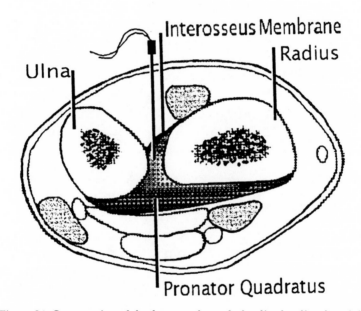

Figure 24. Cross section of the forearm through the distal radio-ulnar joint.

PRONATOR TERES

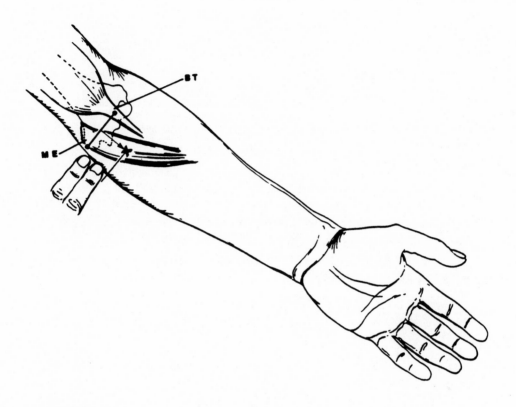

Innervation

Median Nerve, Lateral Cord, Anterior Division, Upper and *Middle* Trunk, C6, *C7*.

Origin

Common tendon from medial epicondyle of humerus and coronoid process of ulna.

Insertion

Lateral surface of radius at mid-shaft.

Position

The forearm fully supinated.

Electrode Insertion (X)

Two fingerbreadths distal to the midpoint of a line connecting the medial epicondyle (ME) and biceps tendon. (BT)

Test Maneuver

Pronation of forearm.

Pitfalls

If the needle electrode is inserted too deeply it will be in the flexor digitorum sublimis; if inserted too ulnarly it will be in the flexor carpi radialis.

Comment

(a) The most proximal muscle innervated by the median nerve.
(b) Common site of entrapment as it is pierced by the median nerve.
(c) May or may not be involved in pronator teres syndrome depending on whether the nerve to the pronator muscle branches proximal to or within the muscle itself.
(d) Also involved in entrapment at the ligament of Struther.

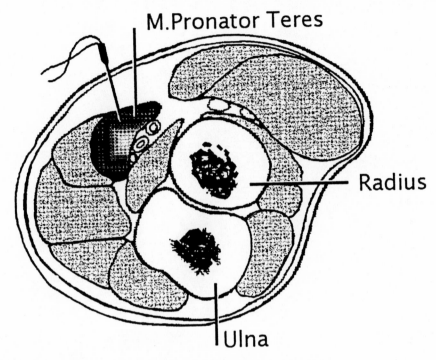

M.Pronator Teres

Radius

Ulna

Figure 25. Cross section of the forearm through distal end of the proximal radio-ulnar joint.

SUPINATOR

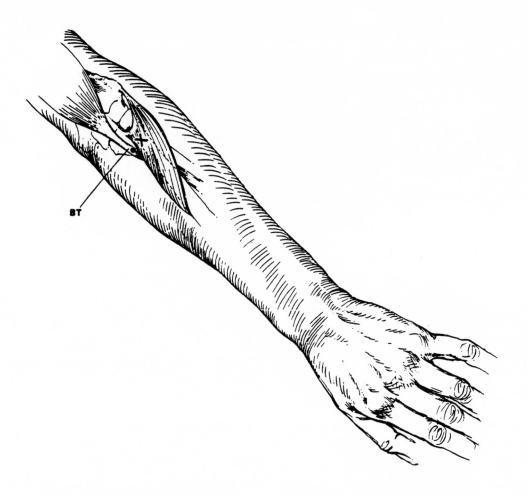

Innervation

Posterior Interosseus Nerve, Radial Nerve, Posterior Cord, Posterior Division, Upper Trunk, C5, *C6.*

Origin

Lateral epicondyle of humerus, radial collateral ligament of elbow, supinator crest of ulna.

Insertion

Dorsal and lateral surfaces of upper third of radial shaft.

Position

The forearm fully pronated.

Electrode Insertion (X)

Just radial to the most distal part of insertion of the biceps tendon (BT). The electrode will travel through the extensor digitorum communis.

Test Maneuver

Supination of forearm.

Pitfalls

If needle electrode is inserted too laterally it will be in the brachioradialis. There is danger of puncturing the radial artery.

Comment

The posterior interosseus nerve passes through an aponeurotic arch (the Arcade of Fröhse) between the two heads of this muscle. When this becomes thickened and tight, it might entrap the nerve.

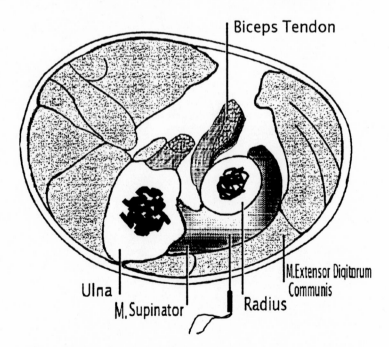

Figure 26. Cross section of the forearm through the proximal third.

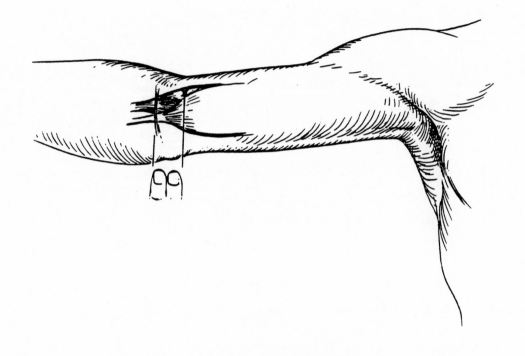

SECTION III
ARM

BICEPS BRACHII

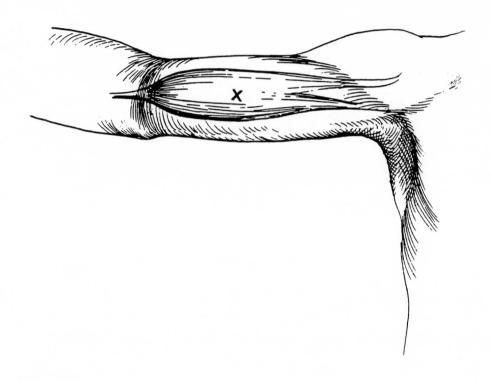

Innervation

Musculocutaneous Nerve, Lateral Cord, Anterior Division, Upper Trunk, *C5, C6.*

Origin

Long Head: From the supraglenoid tuberosity of scapula.
Short Head: From the apex of the coracoid process of the scapula.

Insertion

On the bicipital tuberosity of the radius.

Position

The patient supine with the arm extended.

Electrode Insertion (X)

Into the bulk of the muscle in mid-arm.

Test Maneuver

Flex or supinate forearm.

Pitfalls

If the needle electrode is inserted too deeply it will be in the brachialis.

Comment

(a) Frequently used as recording muscle for musculocutaneous nerve motor conduction study.

(b) Involved in entrapment of musculocutaneous nerve as it courses through the corocobrachialis muscle.

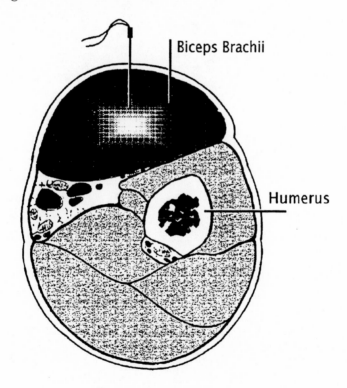

Figure 27. Cross section of the arm through the middle section.

BRACHIALIS

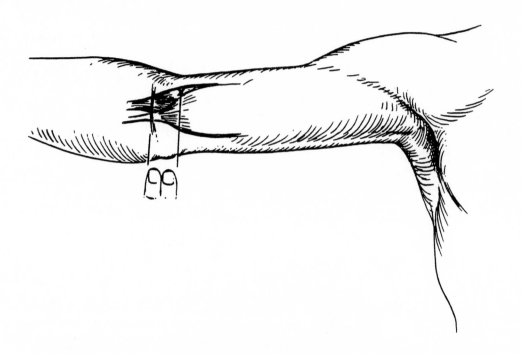

Innervation

Musculocutaneous Nerve, Lateral Cord, Anterior Division, Upper Trunk, *C5*, C6. (Also innervated by a small branch of the radial nerve.)

Origin

From the volar surface of the distal half of the humerus.

Insertion

On the tuberosity of the ulna and volar surface of the coronoid process.

Position

The patient supine with the forearm extended and pronated.

Electrode Insertion (X)

Two fingerbreadths proximal to elbow crease along and just lateral to the tendon and the bulk of the biceps.

Test Maneuver

Flex forearm with the forearm in pronation. The maneuver should be performed against minimal resistance, otherwise the biceps will be activated.

Pitfalls

If the needle electrode is inserted too medially it will be in the biceps.

Comments

(a) Most distal muscle innervated by the musculocutaneous nerve.
(b) Mainly innervated by the musculocutaneous nerve; however, receives a small amount of innervation from the radial nerve.
(c) Involved in musculocutaneous entrapment in the corocobrachialis.

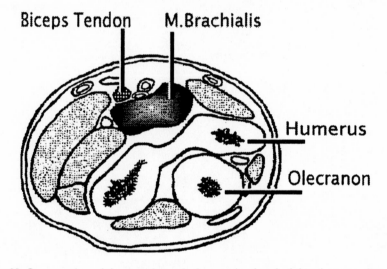

Figure 28. Cross section of the arm through the proximal end of the olecranon fossa.

CORACOBRACHIALIS

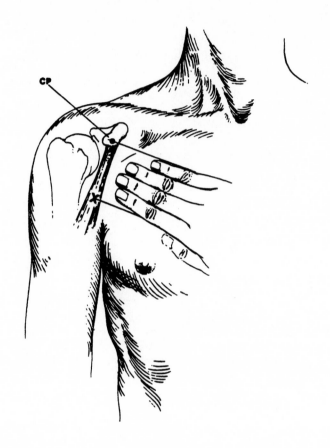

Innervation

Musculocutaneous Nerve, Lateral Cord, Anterior Division, Upper and Middle Trunk, *C6*, C7.

Origin

From the apex of the coracoid process.

Insertion

On the medial border of the humerus opposite the insertion of the deltoid.

Position

Patient supine with arm at side.

Electrode Insertion (X)

Four fingerbreadths distal to the coracoid process (CP) along volar aspect of the arm; insert needle to bone and withdraw.

Test Maneuver

With the elbow flexed to ninety degrees, forward elevation of the arm.

Pitfalls

If the needle electrode is inserted too superficially it will be in the biceps or anterior deltoid; if inserted too laterally it will be in the brachialis.

Comment

(a) The most proximal muscle innervated by the musculocutaneous nerve.
(b) The musculocutaneous nerve may be entrapped as it pierces the coracobrachialis muscle. When this occurs, this muscle is usually spared while the biceps and brachialis may be involved.

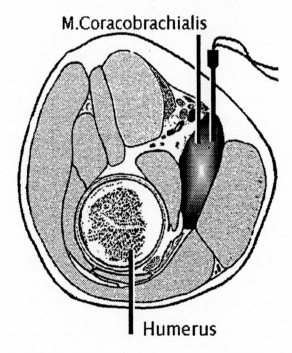

Figure 29. Cross section of the arm through the humeral neck.

TRICEPS

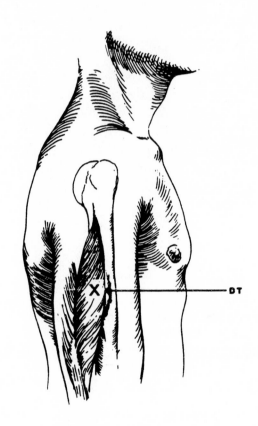

Lateral Head

Innervation

Radial Nerve, Posterior Cord, Posterior Division, Middle and Lower Trunk, *C7, C8,* TI.

Origin

From the dorsal surface of the humerus above the groove for the radial nerve.

Insertion

By common tendon into distal aspect of olecranon process.

Position

Patient prone with arm abducted.

Electrode Insertion (X)

Immediately posterior to the insertion of deltoid or deltoid tubercule (DT).

Test Maneuver

Extension of elbow.

Pitfalls

If the needle electrode is inserted too anteriorly or too proximally it will be in the deltoid.

Comment

Because of its very proximal innervation through the radial nerve, it is almost never involved in "crutch paralysis" or "Saturday night palsy."

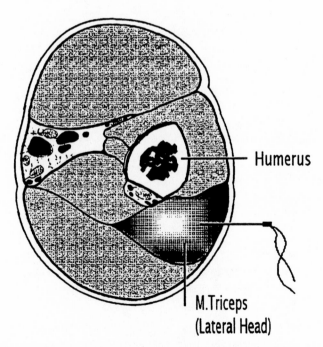

Humerus

M.Triceps
(Lateral Head)

Figure 30. Cross section of the arm through the middle section.

TRICEPS

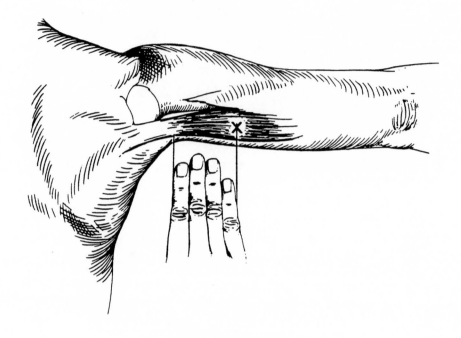

Long Head

Innervation

Radial Nerve, Posterior Cord, Posterior Division, Middle and Lower Trunk, *C7, C8,* TI.

Origin

Infraglenoid tuberosity of the scapula.

Insertion

Via a common tendon, the three heads of the triceps insert on the dorsal aspect of the olecranon process of the ulna.

Position

Patient prone with arm abducted to ninety degrees and elbow flexed over edge of plinth.

Electrode Insertion (X)

Four fingerbreadths distal to the posterior axillary fold.

Test Maneuver

Extension of elbow.

Pitfalls

None.

Comment

Because of its very proximal innervation through the radial nerve, it is almost never involved in "crutch paralysis" or "Saturday night palsy."

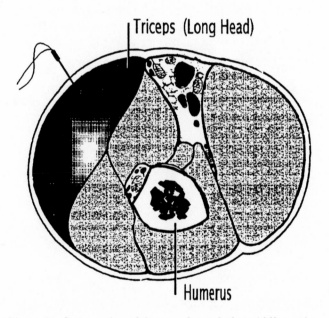

Figure 31. Cross section of the arm through the middle section.

TRICEPS

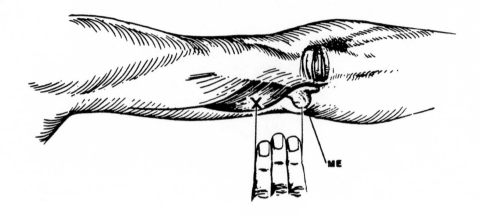

Medial Head

Innervation

Radial Nerve, Posterior Cord, Posterior Division, Middle and Lower Trunk, *C7, C8,* TI.

Origin

From the dorsal surface of the shaft of the humerus below the groove for the radial nerve.

Insertion

By common tendon into olecranon processes.

Position

Patient prone with arm abducted.

Electrode Insertion (X)

Three fingerbreadths proximal to the medial epicondyle (ME) of humerus.

Test Maneuver

Extension of elbow.

Pitfalls

If the needle electrode is inserted too anteriorly it will be in the biceps, and there is also the danger of puncturing the brachial artery.

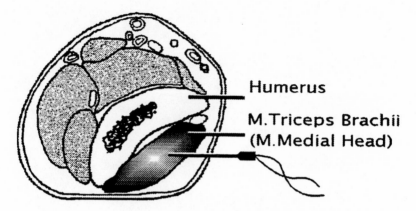

Humerus

M.Triceps Brachii
(M.Medial Head)

Figure 32. Cross section of the arm just proximal to the elbow joint.

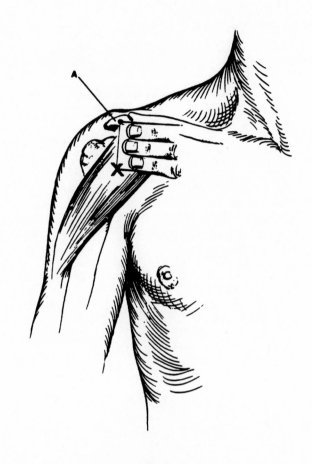

SECTION IV
SHOULDER JOINT

DELTOID, ANTERIOR

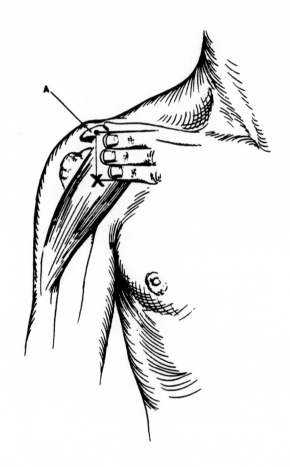

Innervation

Axillary Nerve, Posterior Cord, Posterior Division, Upper Trunk, *C5*, C6.

Origin

Lateral third of the anterior and superior surfaces of the clavicle.

Insertion

Deltoid tubercle of the humerus.

Position

Patient supine with arm at side.

Electrode Insertion (X)

Three fingerbreadths below the anterior margin of the acromion (A).

Test Maneuver

Forward elevation of the arm.

Pitfalls

If the needle electrode is inserted too medially or too deeply it will be in the coracobrachialis.

Comment

(a) Can be used as recording muscle in axillary nerve motor conduction study.
(b) If patient has a history of multiple injections into this muscle, electromyographic findings may be misleading.
(c) Involved in axillary nerve injuries secondary to fracture of surgical neck or glenohumeral joint dislocation.

For cross section, see posterior deltoid, page 95.

DELTOID, MIDDLE

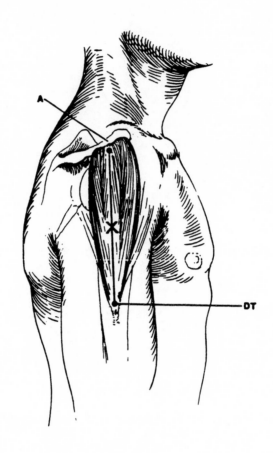

Innervation

Axillary Nerve, Posterior Cord, Posterior Division, Upper Trunk, *C5,* C6.

Origin

Acromion.

Insertion

Deltoid tubercle of the humerus.

Position

Patient supine with arm at side.

Electrode Insertion (X)

Halfway between the tip of the acromion (A) and the deltoid tubercle (DT).

Test Maneuver

Abduction of arm.

Pitfalls

None.

Comment

(a) Generally used as recording muscle in axillary nerve motor conduction study.
(b) If patient has a history of multiple injections into this muscle electromyographic findings may be misleading.
(c) Involved in axillary nerve injuries secondary to fracture of surgical neck or glenohumeral joint dislocation.

For cross section, see posterior deltoid, page 95.

DELTOID, POSTERIOR

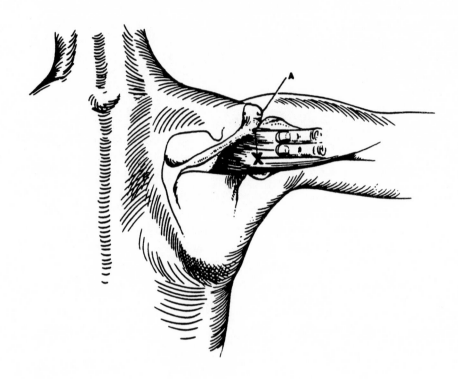

Innervation

Axillary Nerve, Posterior Cord, Posterior Division, Upper Trunk, *C5*, C6.

Origin

The spine of the scapula.

Insertion

Deltoid tubercle of the humerus.

Position

Patient prone with arm abducted to ninety degrees and elbow flexed over edge of plinth.

Electrode Insertion (X)

Two fingerbreadths caudad to posterior margin of the acromion (A).

94

Test Maneuver

Extension of arm.

Pitfalls

If the needle electrode is inserted too medially it will be in the teres minor; if inserted too deeply it will be in the long head of the triceps.

Comment

(a) Can be used as recording muscle in axillary nerve motor conduction study.
(b) If patient has a history of multiple injections into this muscle, electromyographic findings may be misleading.
(c) Involved in axillary nerve injuries secondary to fracture of surgical neck or glenohumeral joint dislocation.

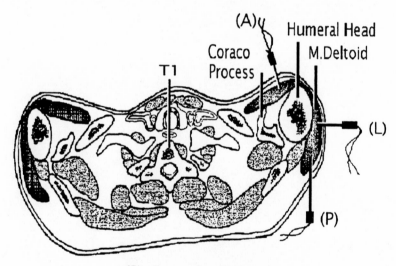

(P): Posterior Deltoid
(L): Lateral Deltoid
(A): Anterior Deltoid

Figure 33. Cross section of the chest at the T1 level.

INFRASPINATUS

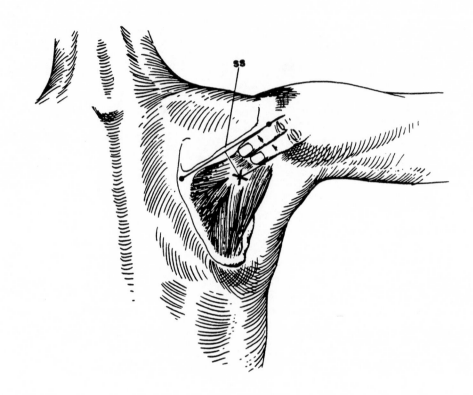

Innervation

Suprascapular Nerve, Upper Trunk, *C5*, C6.

Origin

Infraspinous fossa of scapula.

Insertion

Greater tuberosity of humerus.

Position

Patient prone with arm abducted to ninety degrees and elbow flexed over the edge of plinth.

Electrode Insertion (X)

Insert needle electrode into infraspinous fossa two fingerbreadths below medial portion of spine of scapula (SS).

Test Maneuver

Externally rotate humerus.

Pitfalls

If needle electrode is inserted too superficially it will be in the trapezius; if too laterally it will be in posterior deltoid.

Comment

(a) Used as recording muscle in suprascapular nerve conduction study.
(b) Involved in suprascapular nerve entrapment at the suprascapular notch or at the lateral edge of the spines of the scapular.
(c) Involved in Erb's type of obstetrical palsy.

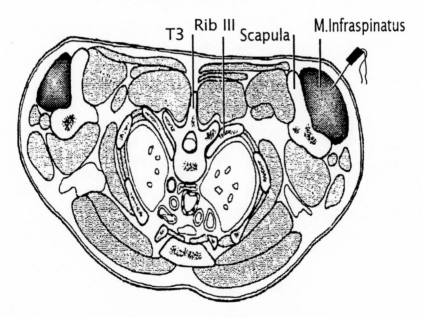

Figure 34. Cross section at the T3 level.

LATISSIMUS DORSI

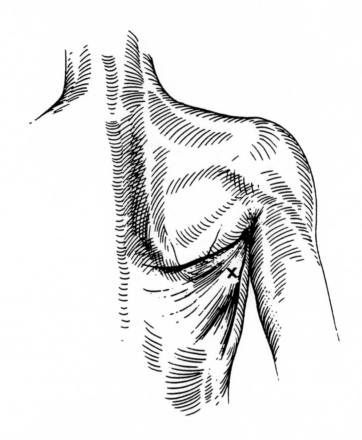

Innervation

Thoracodorsal Nerve, Posterior Cord, Posterior Division, Upper, Middle and Lower Trunk, C6, *C7*, C8.

Origin

Spinous processes of lower thoracic vertebrae, lumbodorsal fascia and posterior crest of ilium.

Insertion

Intertubercular groove of the humerus.

Position

Patient prone with arm at side and palm up.

Electrode Insertion (X)

Three fingerbreadths distal to and along posterior axillary fold.

Test Maneuver

Internally rotate, adduct and extend arm.

Pitfalls

If needle electrode is inserted too medially it will be in the teres major.

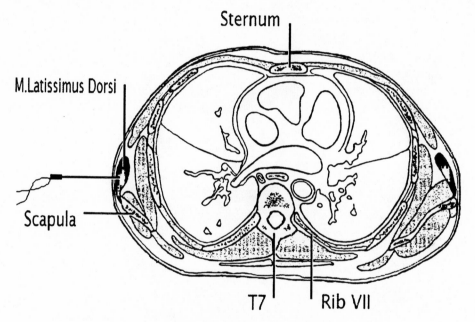

Figure 35. Cross section at T7 level.

PECTORALIS MAJOR

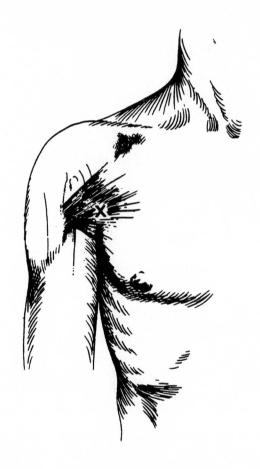

Innervation

Clavicular Portion: Lateral Pectoral Nerve, Lateral Cord, Anterior Division, Upper Trunk, C5, C6.
Sternocostal Portion: Medial Pectoral Nerve, Medial Cord, Anterior Division, Middle and Lower Trunk, C7, C8, TI.

Origin

Medial half of clavicle and anterior surface of sternum and cartilages of the first six ribs.

Insertion

The crest of the greater tubercle of humerus.

Position

Patient supine.

Electrode Insertion (X)

Insert needle electrode into anterior axillary fold.

Test Maneuver

Horizontal adduction of arm.

Pitfalls

If needle electrode is inserted too deeply it will be in the coraco-brachialis; if inserted too laterally it will be in the biceps.

Comment

(a) Innervated by all segments of brachial plexus.
(b) In lateral cord lesions, the clavicular portion is involved. In medial cord lesions, sternocostal position is involved.

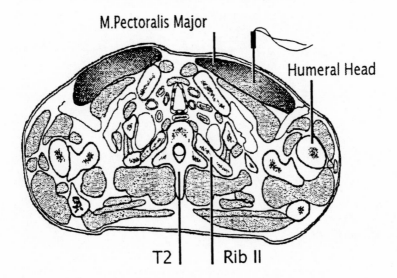

Figure 36. Cross section at T2 level.

SUPRASPINATUS

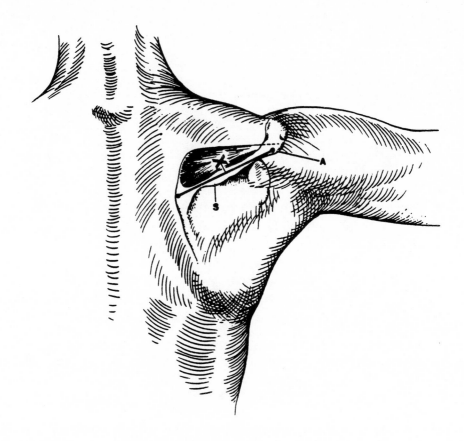

Innervation

Suprascapular Nerve, Upper Trunk, *C5*, C6.

Origins

Supraspinous fossa of scapula.

Insertion

The greater tuberosity of humerus.

Position

Patient prone with arm abducted to ninety degrees and elbow flexed over edge of plinth.

Electrode Insertion (X)

Insert into supraspinous fossa just above middle of spine of scapula (S). The electrode will travel through the midtrapezius muscle.

Test Maneuver

Externally rotate humerus.

Pitfalls

If needle electrode is inserted too superficially it will be in the trapezius.

Comment

(a) Involved in suprascapular nerve entrapment in scapular notch.
(b) Involved in Erb's palsy.

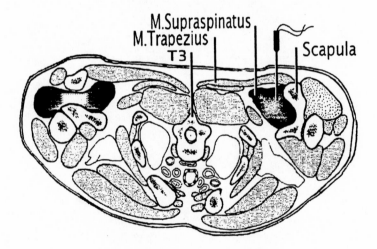

Figure 37. Cross section at T3 level.

TERES MAJOR

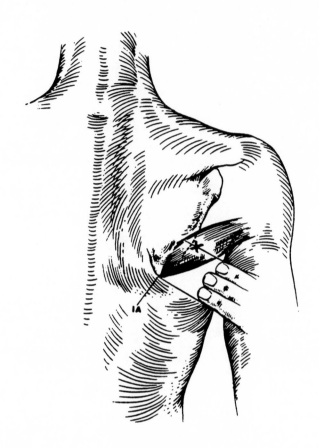

Innervation

Lower Subscapular Nerve, Posterior Cord, Posterior Division, Upper Trunk, *C5, C6.*

Origin

Inferior angle of scapula.

Insertion

The posterior bicipetal ridge.

Position

Patient prone with arm abducted to ninety degrees and elbow flexed over edge of plinth.

Electrode Insertion (X)

Three fingerbreadths above inferior angle (IA) of scapula along the lateral border.

Test Maneuver

Internally rotate humerus.

Pitfalls

If needle electrode is inserted too caudally it will be in the serratus anterior; if inserted too laterally it will be in the latissimus dorsi.

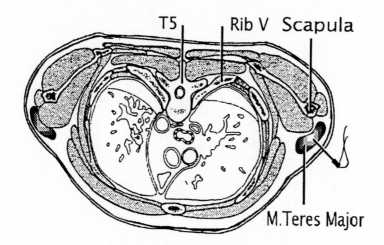

Figure 38. Cross section at T5 level.

TERES MINOR

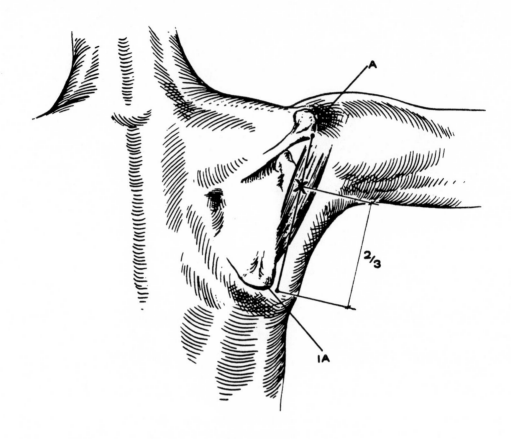

Innervation

Axillary Nerve, Posterior Cord, Posterior Division, Upper Trunk, *C5*, C6.

Origin

Upper two-thirds of axillary border of scapula.

Insertion

The greater tubercle of the humerus.

Position

Patient prone with arm abducted to ninety degrees and elbow flexed over edge of plinth.

Electrode Insertion (X)

Insert one-third of the way between acromion (A) and inferior angle (IA) of scapula along lateral border.

Test Maneuver

Externally rotate humerus.

Pitfalls

If needle electrode is inserted too cephalad, it will be in the supraspinatus; if inserted too caudally, it will be in the teres major; if inserted too superficially, it will be in the trapezius. If inserted too medially, it will be in the infraspinatus.

Comment

(a) It is usually spared in lesions of the axillary nerve secondary to fracture of the surgical neck of the humerus or dislocation of the glenohumeral joint.
(b) Involved in lesions of axillary nerve close to posterior cord.
(c) Involved in Erb's palsy.

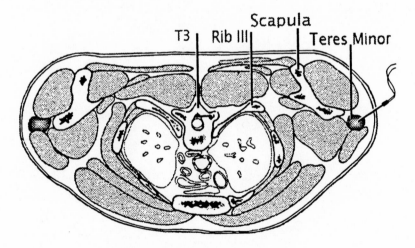

Figure 39. Cross section at T3 level.

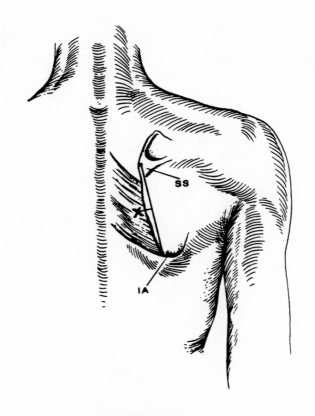

SECTION V
SHOULDER GIRDLE

LEVATOR SCAPULAE

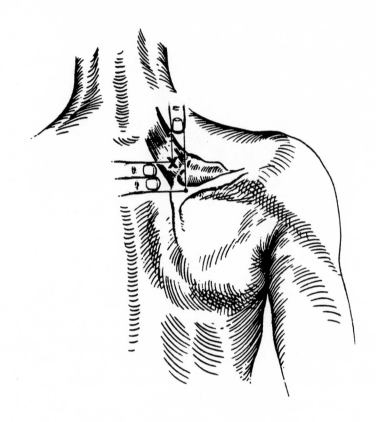

Innervation

Dorsal Scapular Nerve (C5) Plus Twigs From C3, C4.

Origin

Transverse processes of upper four cervical vertebrae.

Insertion

Vertebral border of scapular above root of spine.

Position

Patient prone.

Electrode Insertion (X)

Two fingerbreadths cephalad to the medial angle of scapula and one fingerbreadth medial. The electrode will travel through the upper trapezius.

Test Maneuver

Elevate scapulae.

Pitfalls

If needle electrode is inserted too superficially it will be in the trapezius; if inserted too deeply it will be in the paraspinal muscles.

Comment

This muscle is innervated directly and mainly from C5 root and therefore is an ideal muscle to test integrity of the C5 root.

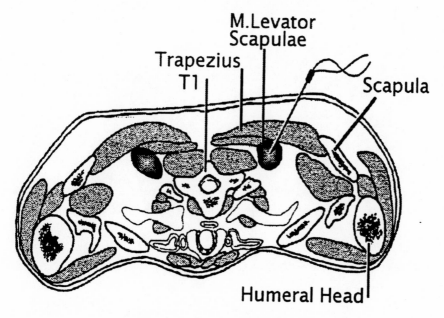

Figure 40. Cross section at T1 level.

PECTORALIS MINOR

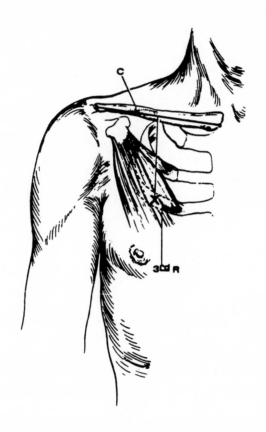

Innervation

Medial and Lateral Pectoral Nerve, Medial and Lateral Cords, Anterior Division, Upper, Middle and Lower Trunks, *C6, C7, C8.*

Origin

Anterior surface of the third to the fifth ribs.

Insertion

Upon the coracoid process of the scapula.

Position

Patient supine.

Electrode Insertion (X)

In midclavicular line insert needle electrode to anterior surface of the third rib (3rd R) and withdraw slightly. The electrode will travel through the pectoralis major.

Test Maneuver

Scapula depression.

Pitfalls

If needle electrode is inserted too superficially it will be in the pectoralis major.

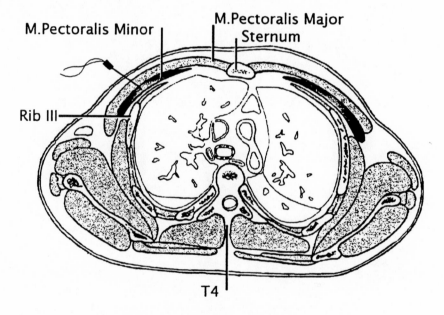

Figure 41. Cross section at T4 level.

RHOMBOIDEUS MAJOR

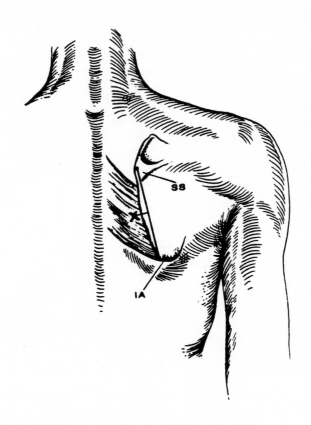

Innervation

Dorsal Scapular Nerve, *C5*.

Origin

Spinous processes of the second to fifth thoracic vertebrae.

Insertion

Vertebral border of scapula: from root of spine of scapula to its inferior angle.

Position

Patient prone with arm internally rotated so that dorsum of hand rests on small of back.

Electrode Insertion (X)

Midway between spine (SS) and inferior angle (IA) of scapula just medial to vertebral border. The electrode will travel through the middle trapezius.

Test Maneuver

Raise hand from small of back.

Pitfalls

If needle electrode is inserted too superficially it will be in the trapezius; if inserted too deeply it will be in the erector spinae muscles.

Comment

Along with the rhomboideus minor, innervated directly and solely from the C5 nerve root; therefore ideal muscles to test for the integrity of the C5 root.

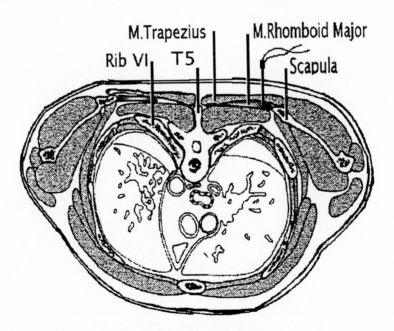

Figure 42. Cross section at T5 level.

RHOMBOIDEUS MINOR

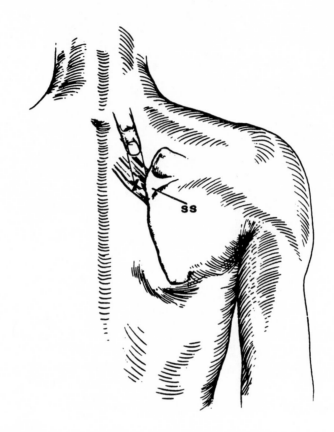

Innervation

Dorsal Scapular Nerve, *C5.*

Origin

Spinous processes of seventh cervical and first thoracic vertebrae.

Insertion

Vertebral border of scapula at the base of the spine of the scapula.

Position

Patient prone with arm internally rotated so that dorsum of hand rests on small of back.

Electrode Insertion (X)

One fingerbreadth medial to vertebral end of scapular spine (SS). The electrode will travel through the upper trapezius.

116

Test Maneuver

Raise hand from small of back.

Pitfalls

If needle electrode is inserted too deeply it will be in the serratus posterior superior.

Comment

See rhomboiseus major.

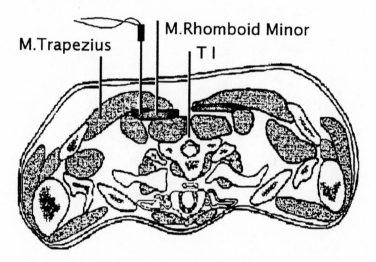

Figure 43. Cross section at T1 level.

SERRATUS ANTERIOR

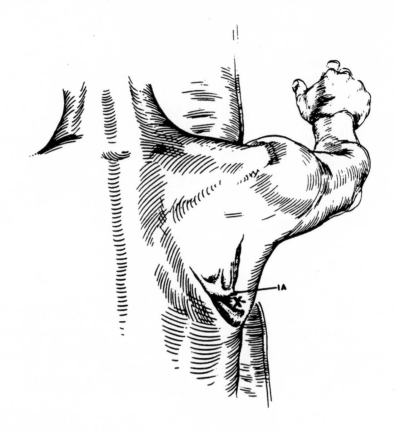

Innervation

Long Thoracic Nerve, *C5, C6, C7.*

Origin

Digitations from anterior surfaces and superior borders of upper nine ribs.

Insertion

Ventral surface of vertebral border of scapula, from superior to inferior angles.

Position

Patient prone with arm dangling over edge of plinth.

Electrode Insertion (X)

Just lateral to inferior angle (IA) of scapula.

Test Maneuver

Patient presses hand against resistance.

Pitfalls

If needle electrode is inserted too superficially it will be in the latissimus dorsi; if inserted too cephalad it will be in the teres major.

Comment

Innervated directly from roots C5, C6, C7 through long thoracic nerve; therefore a good muscle to study when trying to distinguish root from more distal lesions.

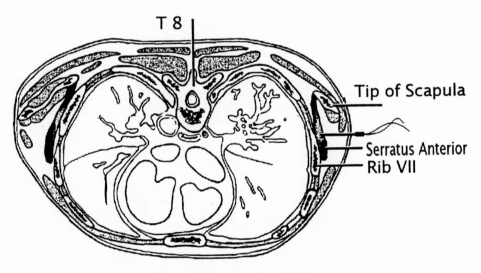

Figure 44. Cross section at T8 level.

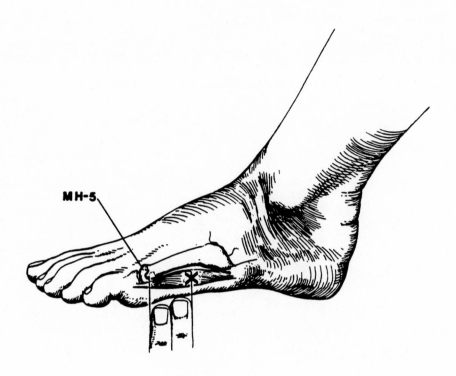

MH-5

SECTION VI
FOOT

ABDUCTOR DIGITI QUINTI

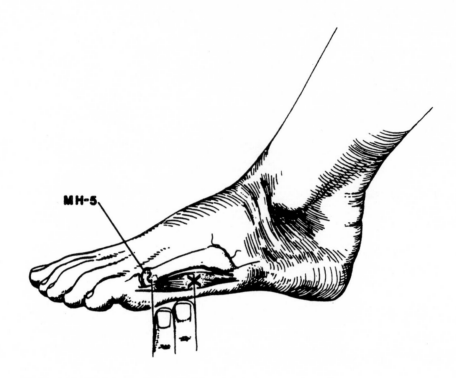

Innervation

Lateral Plantar Nerve, Tibial Nerve, Sciatic Nerve, Ventral Division Sacral Plexus, S1, S2.

Origin

From the lateral process of the tuberosity of the calcaneus.

Insertion

To the lateral side of the base of the proximal phalanx of the fifth toe.

Position

The patient supine.

Electrode Insertion (X)

On the lateral border of the foot, two fingerbreadths proximal to the head of the fifth metatarsal (MH-5).

Test Maneuver

Patient to spread the toes.

Pitfalls

None.

Comment

(a) Commonly involved in—
    1. Peripheral neuropathy secondary to diabetes mellitus
    2. Lateral plantar nerve lesion
    3. Tarsal-tunnel syndrome idiopathic or following ankle fractures
    4. More proximal lesions involving the tibial or sciatic nerve, sacral plexus or S1, S2 roots.
(b) This muscle can be used as recording muscle for the tibial nerve conduction studies; the distal latency will indicate the functional status of the lateral plantar nerve.

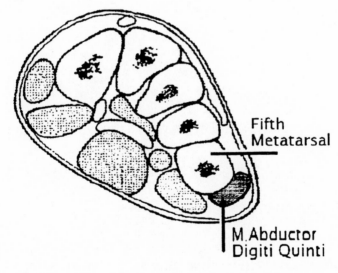

Figure 45. Cross section of the foot at the proximal end of the metatarsal bones.

ABDUCTOR HALLUCIS

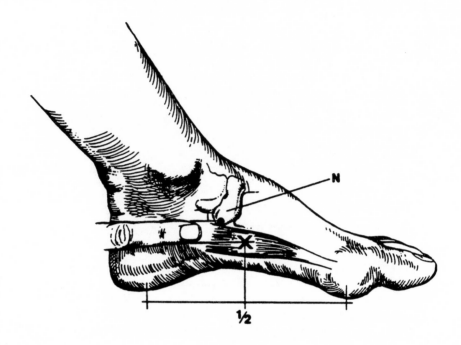

Innervation

Medial Plantar Nerve, Tibial Nerve, Sciatic Nerve, Ventral Division Sacral Plexus, S1–S2.

Origin

From the medial tuberosity of the calcaneus.

Insertion

To the medial side of the base of the proximal phalanx of the great toe.

Position

The patient supine.

Electrode Insertion (X)

One fingerbreadth below the navicular (N) bone on midportion of medial aspect of foot.

Test Maneuver

Patient to spread the toes.

Pitfalls

If the electrode is inserted too distally it will be in the flexor pollicis brevis; if inserted too deeply it will be in the flexor digitorum brevis.

Comment

(a) Commonly involved in—
1. Peripheral neuropathy secondary to diabetes mellitus
2. Medial plantar nerve lesions
3. Tarsal tunnel syndrome, idiopathic or post ankle fracture
4. More proximal lesions involving the tibial or sciatic nerve, sacral plexus or S1, S2 roots.

(b) This muscle can be used as recording muscle for the tibial nerve conduction studies; the distal latency will indicate the functional status of the medial plantar nerve.

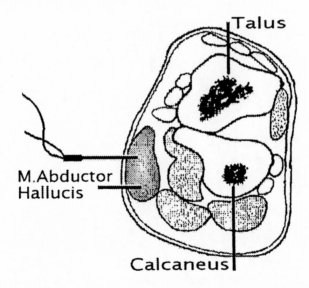

Figure 46. Cross section of the foot through the talocalcaneal joint.

ADDUCTOR HALLUCIS

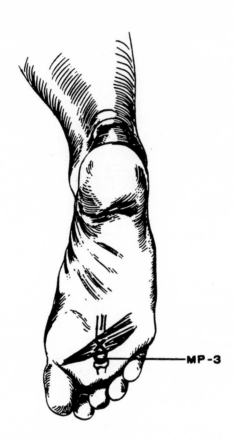

MP-3

Innervation

Lateral Plantar Nerve, Tibial Nerve, Sciatic Nerve, Ventral Division Sacral Plexus, S1, S2.

Origin

From the peroneus longus tendon sheath and adjacent parts of the cuboid and second, third and fourth metatarsal bones (oblique head), and from the capsule of the third, fourth and fifth metatarsalphalangeal joints (transverse head).

Insertion

Into the lateral aspect of the base of the proximal phalanx of the big toe.

126

Position

The patient supine.

Electrode Insertion (X)

For the transverse head only: Insert the electrode just proximal to the third metatarsalphalangeal (MP-3) joint until the metatarsal bone is felt; withdraw the electrode slightly.

Test Maneuver

Passively abduct big toe and ask patient to adduct.

Pitfalls

If the electrode is inserted too superficially it will be in the lumbrical muscle.

Comments

Involved in peripheral neuropathy secondary to diabetes mellitus.

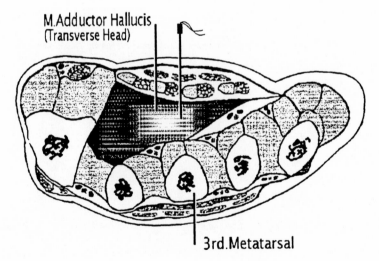

M.Adductor Hallucis (Transverse Head)

3rd.Metatarsal

Figure 47. Cross section of the foot through the distal third of the metatarsal bones.

EXTENSOR DIGITORUM BREVIS

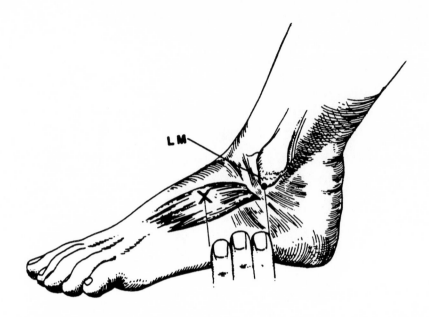

Innervation

Deep Peroneal Nerve, Common Peroneal Nerve, Sciatic Nerve, Dorsal Division Sacral Plexus, L5, S1.

Origin

From the upper and lateral surface of the calcaneus.

Insertion

Into the base of the proximal phalanx of the great toe and the tendon of the extensor digitorum longus of the second, third and fourth toes.

Electrode Insertion (X)

Three fingerbreadths distal to the lower border of the lateral malleolus (LM) parallel to the lateral border of the foot.

Test Maneuver

Patient to extend the toes.

Pitfalls

None.

128

Comment

(a) Last muscle innervated by deep peroneal nerve.
(b) This muscle is used as recording muscle for the common peroneal nerve conduction study.
(c) Involved in—
   1. Lesions of peripheral neuropathy secondary to diabetes mellitus
   2. Deep peroneal nerve lesions
   3. More proximal nerve lesions of common peroneal nerve, sciatic nerve, sacral plexus, or L5, S1 nerve roots.

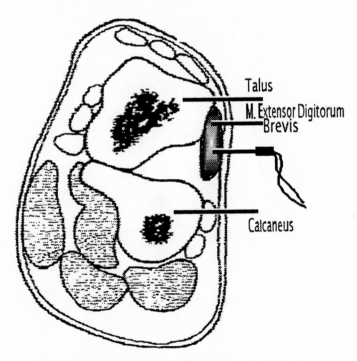

Figure 48. Cross section of the foot through the ankle joint.

FLEXOR DIGITORUM BREVIS

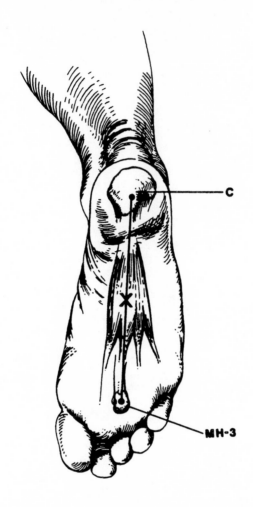

Innervation

Medial Plantar Nerve, Tibial Nerve, Sciatic Nerve, Ventral Division Sacral Plexus, S1, S2.

Origin

From the medial tubercle of the calcaneus and the deep surface of the plantar aponeurosis.

Insertion

Into the plantar surface of the base of the middle phalanx of the second, third, fourth and fifth toes.

Position

Patient supine.

Electrode Insertion (X)

The electrode is inserted midway between the third metatarsal head (MH-3) and the calcaneous (C) to the plantar aponeurosis and then withdrawn slightly.

Test Maneuver

Patient to flex the toes.

Pitfalls

If the electrode is inserted too laterally it will be in the abductor digiti minimi; if inserted too medially it will be in the abductor hallucis brevis; if inserted too deeply it will be in the quadratus plantae.

Comment

Commonly involved in—
(1) Peripheral neuropathy secondary to diabetes mellitus
(2) Medial plantar nerve lesions
(3) Tarsal tunnel syndrome
(4) More proximal lesions involving the tibial nerve, sciatic nerve, sacral plexus or S1, S2 roots.

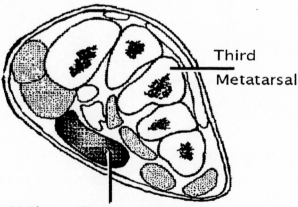

Figure 49. Cross section of the foot through the midportion.

FLEXOR DIGITI QUINTI BREVIS

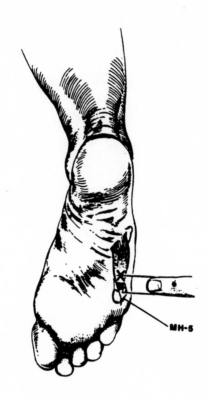

Innervation

Lateral Plantar Nerve, Tibial Nerve, Sciatic Nerve, Ventral Division Sacral Plexus, S1, S2.

Origin

From the sheath of the peroneus longus tendon and the base of the fifth metatarsal bone.

Insertion

In a common tendon with the abductor digit minimi into the lateral side of the base of the proximal phalanx of the little toe.

Position

The patient supine.

132

Electrode Insertion (X)

On the plantar surface of the foot, one fingerbreadth proximal to the fifth metatarsal head (MH-5), the electrode is inserted to the bone and then withdrawn slightly.

Test Maneuver

Patient to flex the metatarsophalangeal joint of the little toe.

Pitfalls

If the electrode is inserted too laterally it will be in the abductor digiti minimi; if inserted too medially it will be in the lumbricals.

Comments

Commonly involved in—
(1) Peripheral neuropathy secondary to diabetes mellitus
(2) Lateral plantar nerve
(3) Tarsal tunnel syndrome
(4) More proximal lesions involving the tibial nerve, sciatic nerve, sacral plexus or S1, S2 roots.

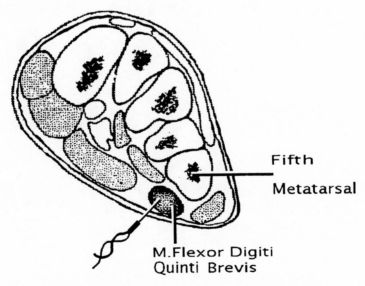

Figure 50. Cross section of the foot through the midportion.

FLEXOR HALLUCIS BREVIS

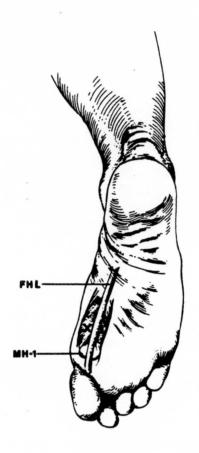

Innervation

Medial Plantar Nerve, Tibial Nerve, Sciatic Nerve, Ventral Division Sacral Plexus, S1, S2.

Origin

The two muscle bellies originate from a tendinous expansion of the tibialis posterior muscle insertion and from the cuneiform and the cuboid.

Insertion

The two tendons end at each side of the base of the proximal phalanx of the big toe, the medial one in a common tendon with that of the abductor, and the lateral one in a common tendon with that of the adductor hallucis brevis.

134

Position

The patient supine.

Electrode Insertion (X)

For medial head only: Proximal and medial to the tendon of the flexor hallucis longus.

Test Maneuver

Patient to flex the metatarsalphalangeal joint of the big toe.

Pitfalls

If the electrode is inserted too laterally it will be in the adductor hallucis; if inserted too medially it will be in the abductor hallucis.

Comment

Commonly involved in—
(1) Peripheral neuropathy secondary to diabetes mellitus
(2) Medial plantar nerve
(3) Tarsal-tunnel syndrome
(4) More proximal lesions involving the tibial nerve, sciatic nerve, sacral plexus or S1, S2 roots.

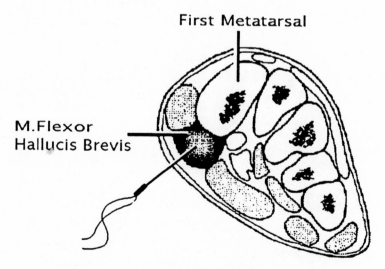

Figure 51. Cross section of the foot through the midportion.

INTEROSSEI*

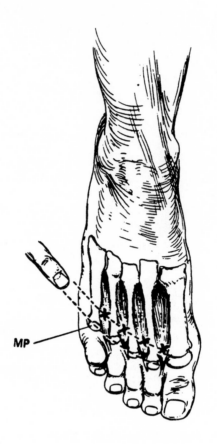

MP

Innervation

Lateral Plantar Nerve, Tibial Nerve, Sciatic Nerve, Sacral Plexus, S1, S2.

Origin

From the shaft of the metatarsal into the base of the proximal phalanges and the dorsal digital expansions.

Position

The patient supine.

Electrode Insertion (X)

The needle electrode is inserted one fingerbreadth proximal to the

---

*It was impossible to differentiate between the dorsal and volar interossei with the needle electrode.

metatarsalphalangeal (MP) joints in the intermetatarsal space. The number of interosseus muscle corresponds to the number of the intermetatarsal space.

Test Maneuver

Spread toes.

Pitfalls

If the needle electrode is inserted too deeply it will be either in the oblique or transverse head of the adductor hallucis.

Comment

This group of muscles is commonly involved in—
(1) Peripheral neuropathy secondary to diabetes mellitus
(2) Lateral plantar nerve lesions
(3) Tarsal-tunnel syndrome
(4) More proximal lesions involving the tibial nerve, sciatic nerve, sacral plexus, or S1, S2 roots.

QUADRATUS PLANTAE

(FLEXOR DIGITORUM ACCESSORIUS)

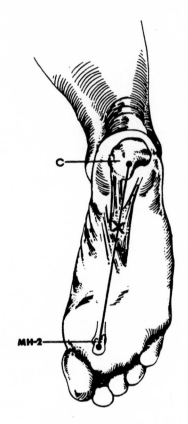

Innervation

Lateral Plantar Nerve, Tibial Nerve, Sciatic Nerve, Ventral Division Sacral Plexus, S1, S2.

Origin

Medial Head: From medial surface of calcaneous.
Lateral Head: From lateral border of the plantar surface of the calcaneous.

Insertion

Into the tendon of the flexor digitorum longus.

Position

The patient supine.

Electrode Insertion (X)

Insert the electrode at the junction of proximal and middle one-third of a line between the tip of the calcaneous (C) and the second metatarsal head (MH-2). Insert deep to bone and withdraw slightly. The electrode will travel through the flexor digitorum brevis muscle.

Test Maneuver

Patient to flex the toes.

Pitfalls

If the electrode is inserted too superficially it will be in the flexor digitorum brevis; if inserted too laterally it will be in the abductor digiti minimi; if inserted too medially it will be in the abductor hallucis brevis.

Comment

Involved in lesions of —
  1. Peripheral neuropathy secondary to diabetes mellitus
  2. Lateral plantar nerve lesions
  3. Tarsal-tunnel syndrome
  4. More proximal lesions of tibial nerve, sciatic nerve, sacral plexus and S1, S2 nerve roots.

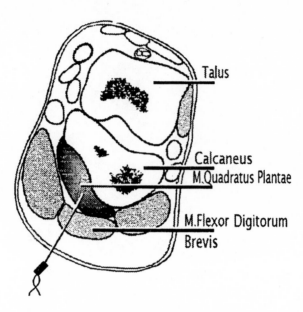

Figure 52. Cross section of the foot through the ankle joint (foot is plantarflexed 45°).

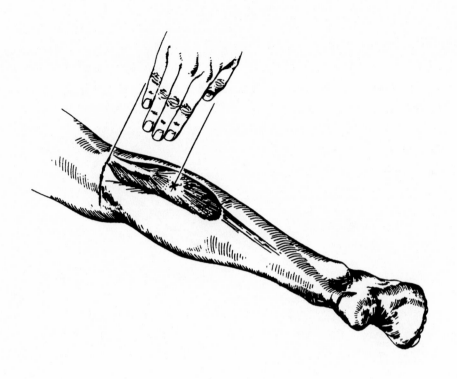

SECTION VII
LEG

EXTENSOR DIGITORUM LONGUS

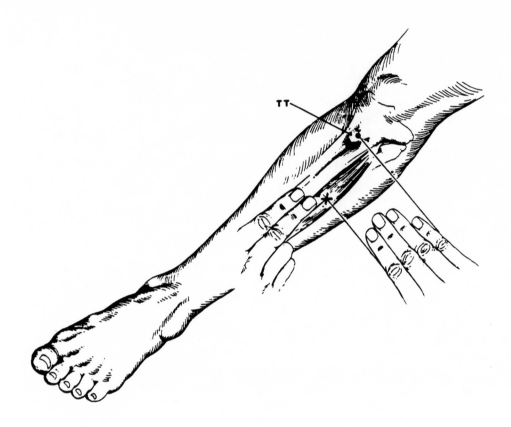

Innervation

Deep Peroneal Nerve, Common Peroneal Nerve, Sciatic Nerve, Posterior Division Sacral Plexus, L5, S1.

Origin

From the lateral condyle of the tibia, the proximal three-fourths of the fibula and the interosseus membrane.

Insertion

Through a common tendon with the lumbricals and the interossei into the dorsum of the middle and distal phalanx of the four lateral toes.

Position

The patient supine.

142

Electrode Insertion (X)

Four fingerbreadths distal to the tibial tubercle (TT) and two finger-breadths lateral to the tibial crest, the electrode is inserted through the tibialis anterior about one inch.

Test Maneuver

Patient to extend the four lateral toes.

Pitfalls

If the electrode is inserted too anteriorly it will be in the tibialis anterior; if inserted too laterally it will be in the peroneus longus.

Comment

Involved in—
1. Anterior compartment syndrome
2. Lesions of the deep peroneal nerve
3. Common peroneal nerve
4. Sciatic nerve
5. Sacral plexus.

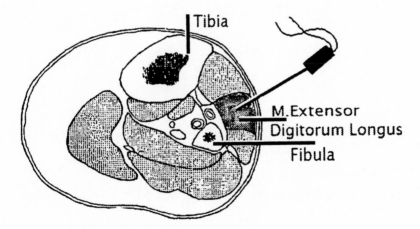

Figure 53. Cross section of the leg through the junction of the upper and middle third.

EXTENSOR HALLUCIS LONGUS

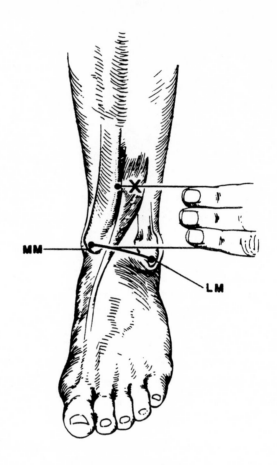

Innervation

Deep Peroneal Nerve, Common Peroneal Nerve, Sciatic Nerve, Posterior Division Sacral Plexus, L5, *S1.*

Origin

From the midportion of the shaft of the fibula.

Insertion

Into the distal phalanx of the great toe.

Position

The patient supine.

Electrode Insertion (X)

Three fingerbreadths above the bimalleolar line (MM–LM) of the ankle just lateral to the crest of the tibia.

Test Maneuver

Patient to extend the big toe.

Pitfalls

If the electrode is inserted too superficially and too proximally it will be in the tibialis anterior; if inserted too laterally it will be in the peroneus tertius.

Comment

Involved in—
1. Anterior compartment syndrome
2. Lesion of the deep peroneal nerve
3. Common peroneal nerve
4. Sciatic nerve
5. Sacral plexus
6. L5, S1 root lesions.

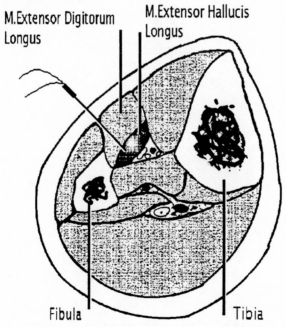

M.Extensor Digitorum Longus

M.Extensor Hallucis Longus

Fibula

Tibia

Figure 54. Cross section of the leg through the junction of the middle and lower third.

FLEXOR DIGITORUM LONGUS

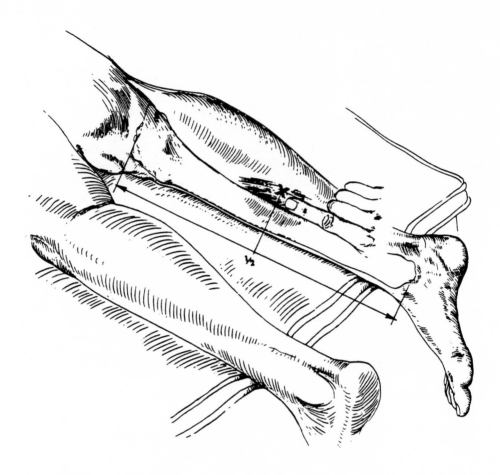

Innervation

Tibial Nerve, Sciatic Nerve, Ventral Division Sacral Plexus, *L5, S1,* S2.

Origin

From the body of the tibia below the popliteal line.

Insertion

Into the base of the distal phalanges of the second, third, fourth and fifth toe.

Position

The patient prone.

Electrode Insertion (X)

Palpate the medial edge of tibia at midshaft and insert electrode just posterior to it.

Test Maneuver

Patient to flex the toes, without flexing the ankle.

Pitfalls

If the electrode is inserted too superficially it will be in the soleus; if inserted too deeply it will be in the tibialis posterior.

Comment

Involved in lesions of:
1. The tibial nerve
2. Sciatic nerve
3. Sacral plexus
4. L5, S1, S2 roots.

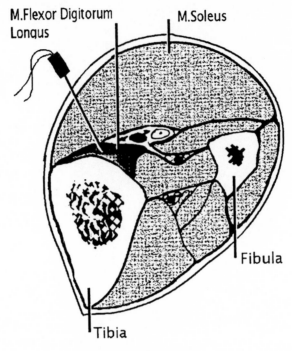

Figure 55. Cross section of the leg through the junction of the middle and lower third.

FLEXOR HALLUCIS LONGUS

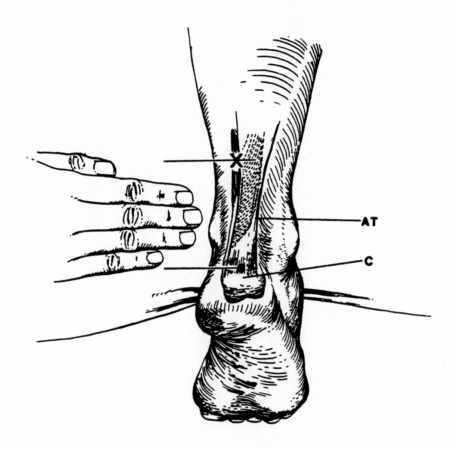

Innervation

Tibial Nerve, Sciatic Nerve, Ventral Division Sacral Plexus, L5, S1, S2.

Origin

From the inferior two-thirds of the posterior surface of body of the fibula and the interosseus membrane.

Insertion

Into the base of the distal phalanx of the great toe.

Position

The patient prone.

Electrode Insertion (X)

Insert the electrode obliquely five fingerbreadths above the insertion of the Achilles tendon (AT) and anterior to the medial border of this tendon towards the tibia.

Test Maneuver

Patient to flex the big toe, keeping the ankle and the small toes relaxed.

Pitfalls

If the electrode is inserted too deeply it will be in the tibialis posterior; if inserted too anteriorly it will be in the flexor digitorum longus; if inserted too superficially it will be in the soleus.

Comment

Involved in lesions of:
1. Tibial nerve
2. Sciatic nerve
3. Sacral plexus
4. L5, S1, S2 roots.

M.Flexor Hallucis Longus   **Calcaneal Tendon**

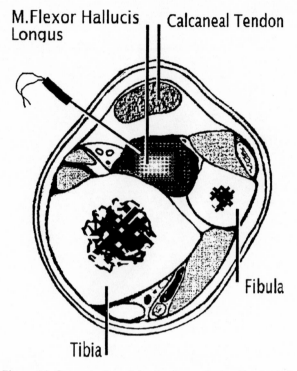

Fibula

Tibia

Figure 56. Cross section of the leg through the distal third.

GASTROCNEMIUS: LATERAL HEAD

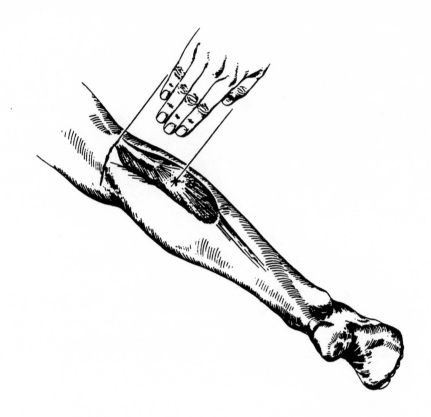

Innervation

Tibial Nerve, Sciatic Nerve, Ventral Division Sacral Plexus, S1, S2.

Origin

From the lateral femoral condyle.

Insertion

Into the calcaneous, through the Achille's tendon.

Position

The patient prone with feet over edge of plinth.

Electrode Insertion (X)

One handbreadth below the popliteal crease on the lateral mass of the calf.

Test Maneuver

Patient to plantar flex the foot with the knee extended.

Pitfalls

If the electrode is inserted too deeply it will be in the soleus.

Comment

Involved in lesions of:
1. Tibial nerve
2. Sciatic nerve
3. Sacral plexus
4. L5, S1, S2 roots.

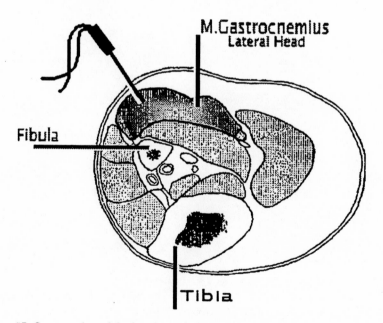

Figure 57. Cross section of the leg through the junction of the upper and middle third.

GASTROCNEMIUS: MEDIAL HEAD

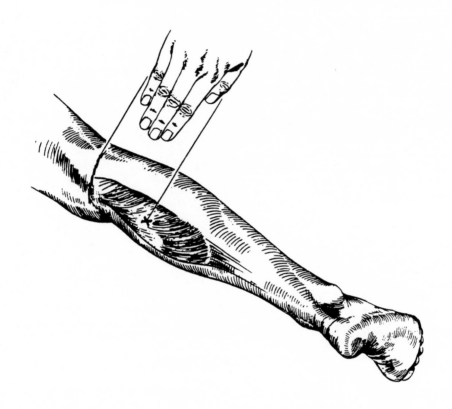

Innervation

Tibial Nerve, Sciatic Nerve, Ventral Division Sacral Plexus, S1, S2.

Origin

From the medial femoral condyle.

Insertion

Into the calcaneous, through the Achille's tendon.

Position

The patient prone with feet over edge of plinth.

Electrode Insertion (X)

One hand breadth below the popliteal crease on the medial mass of the calf.

Test Maneuver

Patient to plantar flex the foot with the knee extended.

Pitfalls

If the electrode is inserted too deeply it will be in the flexor digitorum longus.

Comment

Involved in lesions of:
1. Tibial nerve
2. Sciatic nerve
3. Sacral plexus
4. L5, S1, S2 roots.

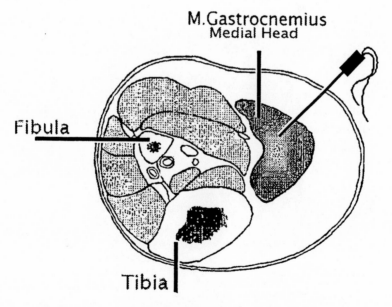

Figure 58. Cross section of the leg through the junction of the upper and middle third.

PERONEUS BREVIS

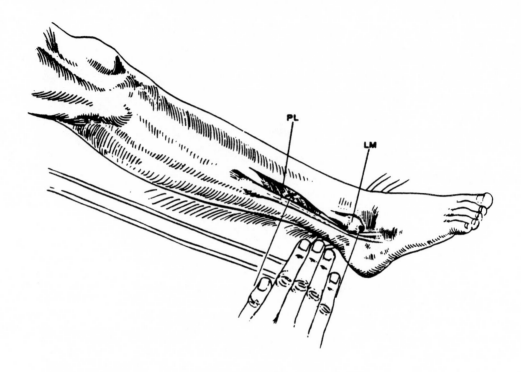

Innervation

Superficial Peroneal Nerve, Common Peroneal Nerve, Sciatic Nerve, Posterior Division Sacral Plexus, *L5, S1,* S2.

Origin

From the lower two-thirds of the fibula.

Insertion

Into the base of the fifth metatarsal head.

Position

The patient supine.

Electrode Insertion (X)

One handbreadth proximal to the lateral malleolus (LM) and anterior to the peroneus longus (PL) tendon.

Test Maneuver

Patient to plantar flex and evert the foot.

Pitfalls

If the electrode is inserted too proximally it will be in the peroneus longus; if inserted too anteriorly it will be either in the peroneus tertius or in the extensor digitorum longus.

Comment

(a) Can be used as recording muscle when the superficial peroneal nerve is to be studied.
(b) Involved in lesions of:
    1. Superficial peroneal nerve
    2. Common peroneal nerve
    3. Sciatic nerve
    4. Sacral plexus
    5. L5, S1 roots.

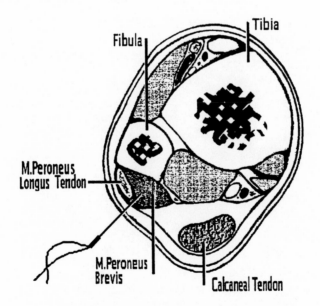

Figure 59. Cross section of the leg through the distal third.

PERONEUS LONGUS

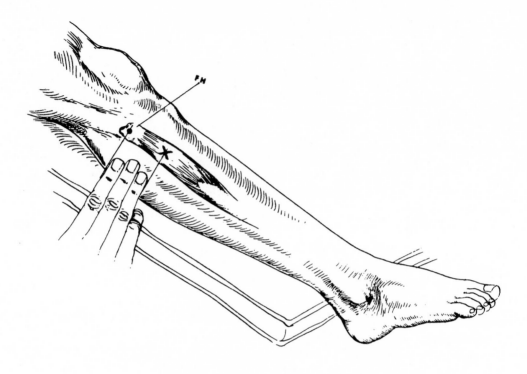

Innervation

Superficial Peroneal Nerve, Common Peroneal Nerve, Sciatic Nerve, Posterior Division Sacral Plexus, *L5, S1,* S2.

Origin

From the fibular head and from the proximal two-thirds of the fibula.

Insertion

Into the base of the first metatarsal and the first cuneiform.

Position

The patient supine.

Electrode Insertion (X)

Three fingerbreadths below the fibular head (FH) directed toward the lateral aspect of the fibula.

Test Maneuver

Patient to plantar flex and evert the foot.

Pitfalls

If the electrode is inserted too posteriorly it will be in the soleus; if inserted too anteriorly it will be in the extensor digitorum longus.

Comment

This muscle is involved in lesions of:
1. Superficial peroneal nerve
2. Common peroneal nerve
3. Sciatic nerve
4. Sacral plexus
5. L5, S1 roots.

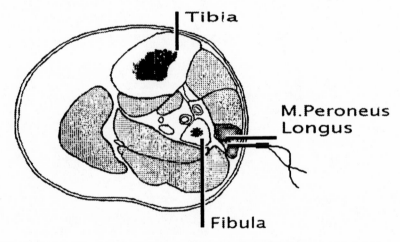

Figure 60. Cross section of the leg through the junction of the upper and middle third.

PERONEUS TERTIUS

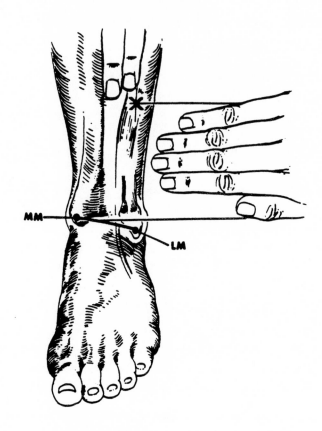

Innervation

Deep Peroneal Nerve, Common Peroneal Nerve, Sciatic Nerve, Posterior Division Sacral Plexus, L5, S1.

Origin

From the lower one-third of the fibula.

Insertion

Into the base of the fifth metatarsal head.

Position

The patient supine.

Electrode Insertion (X)

One handbreadth above bimalleolar line (MM–LM) of the ankle and two fingerbreadths lateral to the tibia.

Test Maneuver

Patient to dorsiflex and evert the foot.

Pitfalls

If the electrode is inserted too medially it will be in the extensor hallucis longus; if inserted too proximally it will be in the tibialis anterior or the extensor digitorum longus.

Comment

(a) This is the only peroneal muscle located in the anterior compartment of the leg. Therefore, it becomes involved in anterior compartment syndrome.
(b) This muscle may be considered as part of the extensor digitorum longus (its fifth tendon).
(c) It is involved in lesions of:
    1. Deep peroneal nerve
    2. Common peroneal nerve
    3. Sciatic nerve
    4. Sacral plexus
    5. L5, S1.

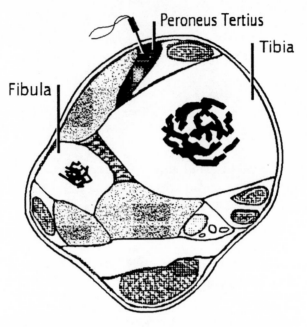

Figure 61. Cross section of the leg through the distal third.

POPLITEUS

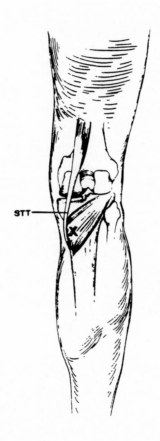

Innervation

Tibial Nerve, Sciatic Nerve, Anterior Division Sacral Plexus, *L5*, S1.

Origin

From the fibrous capsule of the knee joint on the side of the lateral condyle of the femur.

Insertion

Into the triangular area of the tibia above the soleal line.

Position

The patient prone with the knee fully extended.

163

Electrode Insertion (X)

The needle electrode is inserted laterally to the insertion of the semitendinosus tendon (STT).

Test Maneuver

Flex and internally rotate tibia.

Pitfalls

· If the needle electrode is inserted either too distally or too superficially it will be in the gastrocnemius.

Comment

Involved in lesions of:
1. High tibial nerve
2. Sciatic nerve
3. Sacral plexus
4. L5, S1 roots.

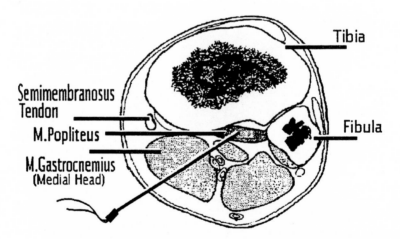

Figure 62. Cross section of the leg through the fibula head.

SOLEUS

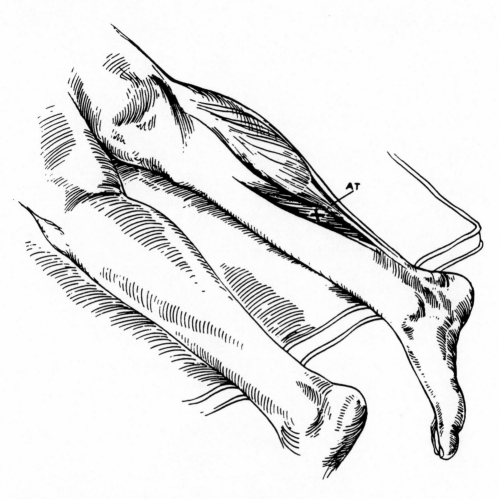

Innervation

Tibial Nerve, Sciatic Nerve, Anterior Division Sacral Plexus, L5, *S1, S2.*

Origin

From the head and the proximal portion of the body of the fibula and the middle one-third of the medial border of the tibia.

Insertion

Through the Achille's tendon, on calcaneous bone.

Electrode Insertion (X)

Insert the electrode distal to the belly of the gastrocnemius muscle, medial and anterior to the achilles tendon (AT).

Test Maneuver

Patient to plantar flex foot with knee flexed.

Pitfalls

If electrode is inserted too superficially it will be in the gastrocnemius.

Comments

(a) Muscle most commonly used to study the "H" reflex.
(b) This muscle is involved in lesions of:
    1. Tibial nerve
    2. Sciatic nerve
    3. Sacral plexus
    4. S1, S2 roots.

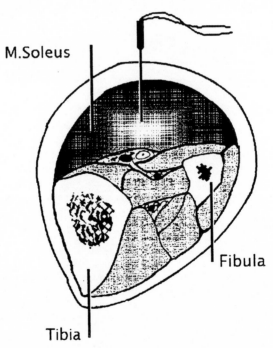

Figure 63. Cross section of the leg through the midportion.

TIBIALIS ANTERIOR

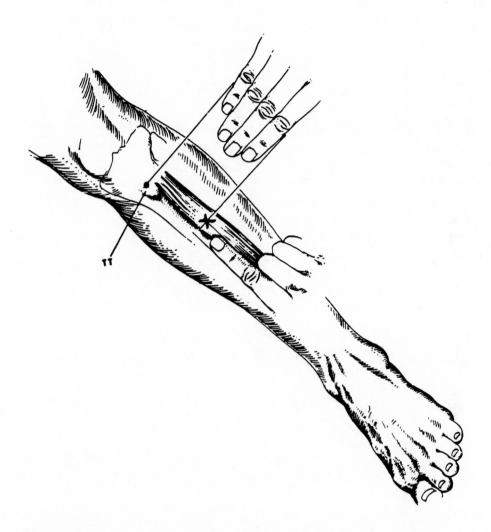

Innervation

Deep Peroneal Nerve, Common Peroneal Nerve, Sciatic Nerve, Posterior Division Sacral Plexus, L4, L5.

Origin

From the lateral condyle and the proximal two-thirds of the shaft of the tibia.

Insertion

On the first cuneiform and the base of the first metatarsal.

Position

The patient supine.

Electrode Insertion (X)

Four fingerbreadths below the tibial tuberosity (TT) and one finger-breadth lateral to the tibial crest.

Test Maneuver

Patient to dorsiflex the foot.

Pitfalls

If the electrode is inserted too laterally and too deeply it will be in the extensor digitorum communis.

Comments

    (a) First muscle innervated by the deep peroneal nerve.
    (b) Involved in lesions of:
        1. Deep peroneal nerve
        2. Common peroneal nerve
        3. Sciatic nerve
        4. Sacral plexus
        5. L4, L5 roots.

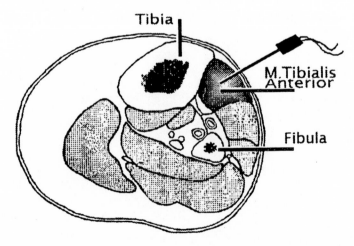

Figure 64. Cross section of the leg through the junction of the upper and middle third.

TIBIALIS POSTERIOR

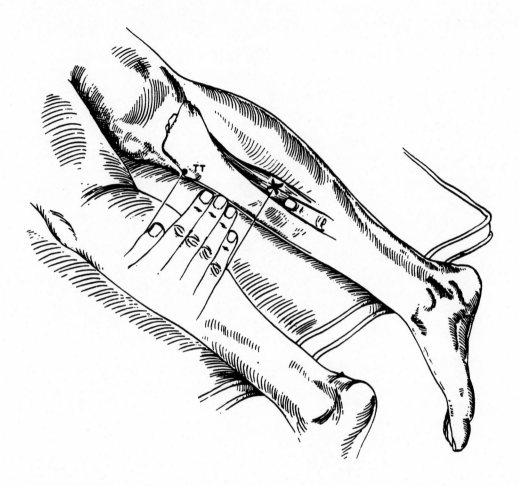

Innervation

Tibial Nerve, Sciatic Nerve, Anterior Division Sacral Plexus, L5, S1.

Origin

From the interosseus membrane, the posterior surface of the body of the tibia and the upper two-thirds of the medial surface of the fibula.

Insertion

On the tuberosity of the navicula bone and through fibrous expansions into the sustentaculumtali and the calcaneous.

Position

The patient prone with feet over edge of plinth, thigh internally rotated.

Electrode Insertion (X)

One handbreadth distal to the tibial tuberosity (TT) and one fingerbreadth off the medial edge of the tibia. The electrode is directly obliquely through the soleus and flexor digitorum longus, just posterior to the tibia.

Test Maneuver

Patient to invert foot in plantar flexion.

Pitfalls

If the electrode is inserted too superficially it will be in the soleus or flexor digitorum longus; if inserted too deeply it will be in the tibialis anterior.

Comment

Involved in lesions of:
1. Tibial nerve
2. Sciatic nerve
3. Sacral plexus
4. L5, S1 root.

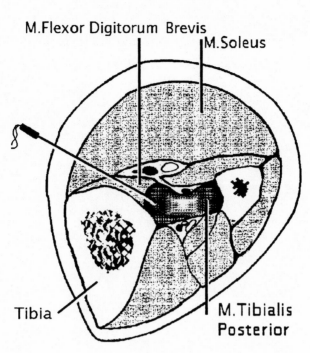

Figure 65. Cross section of the leg through the midportion.

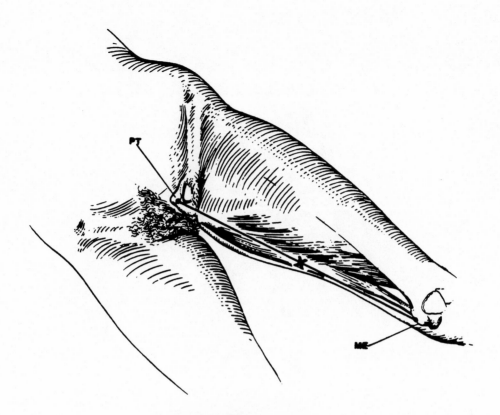

SECTION VIII
THIGH

ADDUCTOR BREVIS

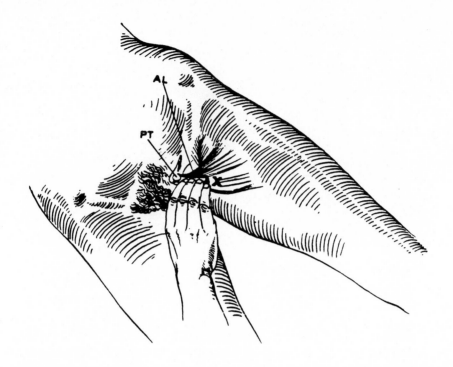

Innervation

Obturator Nerve, Anterior Division Lumbar Plexus, L2, L3, L4.

Origin

From the inferior ramus of the pubis.

Insertion

To a line below the lesser trochanter of the femur.

Position

The patient supine with both lower extremities abducted fifteen degrees.

Electrode Insertion (X)

Palpate the tendon of adductor longus (AL) arising from pubic tubercle (PT) and insert electrode four fingerbreadths distal to tubercle through the adductor longus muscle to about two inches.

Text Maneuver

Patient to adduct the limb.

Pitfalls

If the electrode is inserted too superficially it will be in the adductor longus (laterally) or in the gracilis (medially); if inserted too medially it will be in the adductor magnus.

Comment

Involved in—
1. Anterior branch of the obturator nerve lesions
2. Obturator nerve lesions
3. Anterior division of the lumbar plexus lesions
4. L2, L3, L4 roots lesions
5. Landmark for obturator nerve block. Anterior branch lies on ventral surface of muscle, posterior branch lies on the posterial surface.

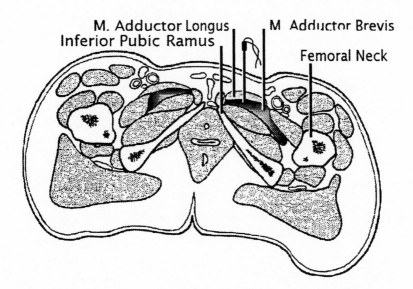

Figure 66. Cross section of the pelvis through the inferior pubic ramus.

ADDUCTOR LONGUS

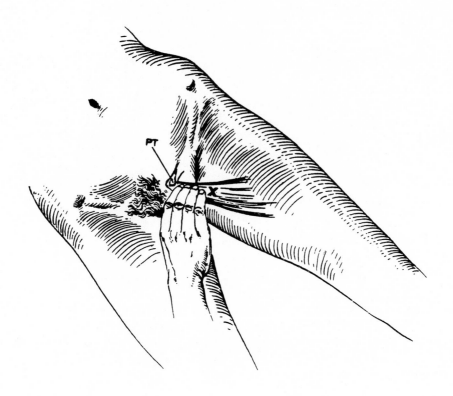

Innervation

Obturator Nerve, Anterior Division Lumbar Plexus, *L2, L3, L4.*

Origin

From the pubic tubercle.

Insertion

Into the linea aspera, between the adductor magnus and the vastus medialis.

Position

The patient supine with both lower extremities abducted fifteen degrees.

Electrode Insertion (X)

Palpate the tendon arising from the pubic tubercle (PT) and insert the electrode four fingerbreadths distal to the pubic tubercle into the muscle belly.

Test Maneuver

Patient to adduct limb.

Pitfalls

If the electrode is inserted too medially it will be in the gracilis; if inserted too laterally it will be in the sartorius.

Comment

Involved in—
1. Anterior branch of the obturator nerve lesions
2. Obturator nerve lesions
3. Anterior division of the lumbar plexus lesions
4. L2, L3, L4 roots lesions.

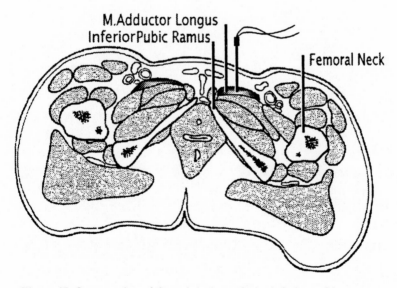

Figure 67. Cross section of the pelvis through the inferior pubic ramus.

ADDUCTOR MAGNUS

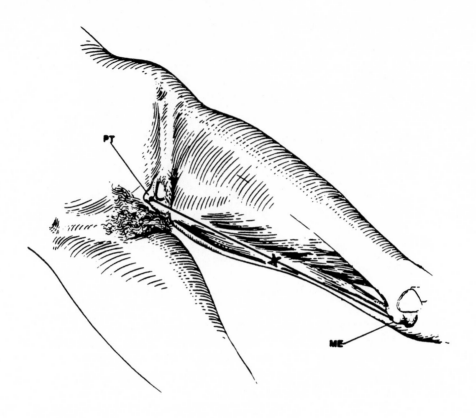

Innervation

Obturator Nerve, Anterior Division Lumbar Plexus, L2, L3, L4, L5.
Also Fibers from sciatic nerve L4, L5.

Origin

From the inferior ramus of the pubis and ischium and the tuberosity
of the ischium.

Insertion

Into the linea aspera and the adductor tubercle of the femur.

Position

The patient supine with both lower extremities abducted fifteen degrees
and externally rotated.

Electrode Insertion (X)

Midway between the medial femoral epicondyle (ME) and the pubic tubercle (PT).

Test Maneuver

Patient to adduct the thigh.

Pitfalls

If the electrode is too superficial it will be in the gracilis; if inserted too laterally it will be in the sartorius; and if inserted too proximally it will be in the adductor longus.

Comments

(a) Partially involved in—
    1. Posterior branch of the obturator nerve*
    2. Obturator nerve lesions
    3. Anterior division of the lumbar plexus
    4. L2, L3, L4 roots lesions.
(b) Also involved in—
    1. High lesions of the sciatic nerve
    2. Anterior divisions of the upper portion of the sacral plexus
    3. L4, L5 roots lesions.

---

*Morphologically the superficial portion of the muscle is considered to be part of the hamstrings muscle group. This accounts for its innervation through the sciatic nerve.

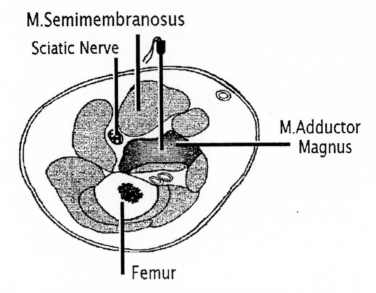

M.Semimembranosus

Sciatic Nerve

M.Adductor
Magnus

Femur

Figure 68. Cross section of the thigh through the middle and distal third.

BICEPS FEMORIS: LONG HEAD

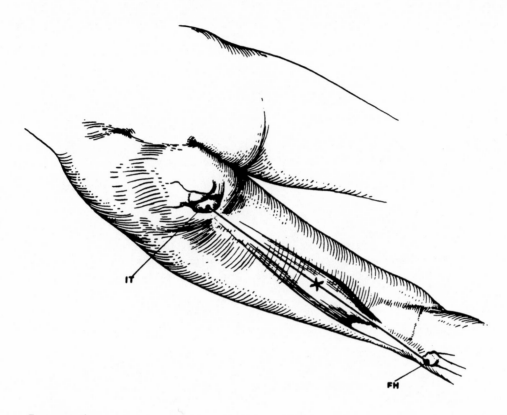

Innervation

Sciatic Nerve (Tibial Portion), Anterior Division, Sacral Plexus, L5, *S1.*

Origin

From the ischial tuberosity.

Insertion

Into the head of the fibula.

Position

The patient prone.

Electrode Insertion (X)

Insert the electrode at the midpoint of a line between the fibula head (FH) and the ischial tuberosity (IT).

Test Maneuver

Patient to flex the knee.

Pitfalls

None.

Comment

Involved in lesions of—
1. Sciatic nerve
2. Anterior division of the sacral plexus
3. L5, S1 roots lesion.

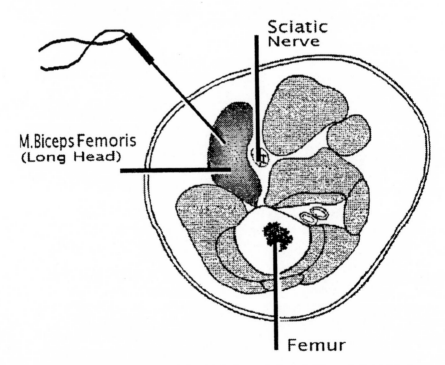

Figure 69. Cross section of the thigh through the middle and distal third.

BICEPS FEMORIS: SHORT HEAD

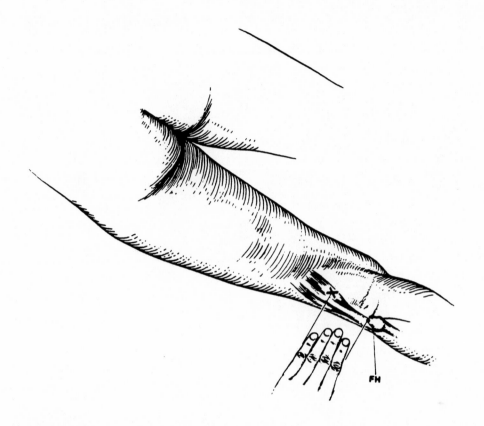

Innervation

Sciatic Nerve, (Peroneal Division) Posterior Division, Sacral Plexus, L5, *S1, S2.*

Origin

From the lateral lip of the linea aspera and the upper part of the lateral supracondylar line.

Insertion

Into the head of the fibula and the lateral condyle of the tibia.

Position

The patient prone with the knee flexed to ninety degrees.

Electrode Insertion (X)

Palpate the tendon of the long head of the biceps; grasp it with the fingertips; insert the electrode just medial to it, four fingerbreadths proximal to the fibular head (FH).

Test Maneuver

Patient to flex the knee.

Pitfalls

If the electrode is inserted too medially it will be in the semimembranosus; if inserted too laterally it will be in the long head of the biceps femoris.

Comment:

(a) Involved in lesions of —
  1. Sciatic Nerve
  2. Anterior division of the sacral plexus
  3. L5, S1 roots lesion.
(b) Only muscle above the knee innervated by the peroneal division of the sciatic nerve.

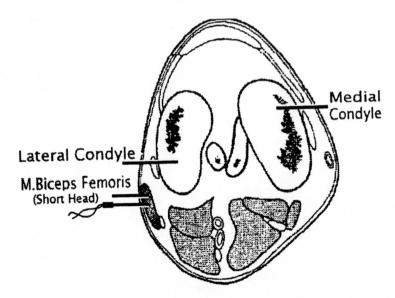

Figure 70. Cross section of the thigh through the upper portion of the knee joint.

GRACILIS

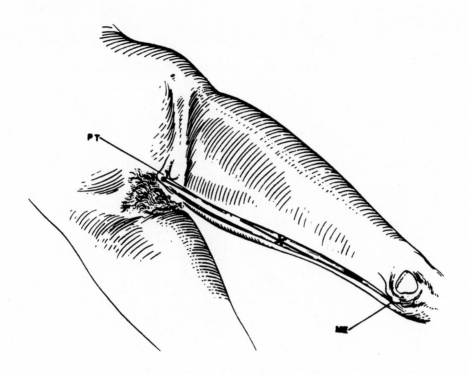

Innervation

Obturator Nerve, Anterior Division Lumbar Plexus, *L2, L3,* L4.

Origin

From the lower half of the symphysis pubis and the pubic arch.

Insertion

Into the medial surface of the tibia below the condyle.

Electrode Insertion (X)

Insert the electrode to a maximum depth of one-half inch at a point midway between the pubic tubercle (PT) and the medial femoral epicondyle (ME).

Test Maneuver

Patient to adduct the thigh and flex the knee.

Pitfall

If the electrode is inserted too deeply it will be in the adductor magnus; if inserted too laterally it will be in the adductor longus.

Comment

Involved in lesions of—
1. Anterior branch of the obturator nerve
2. Obturator for nerve
3. Anterior division of the lumbar plexus
4. L2, L3, L4 roots lesions.

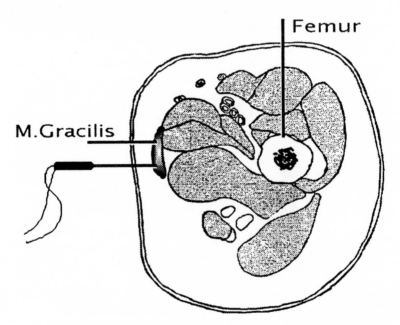

Figure 71. Cross section of the thigh through the junction of the upper and middle third.

ILIOPSOAS

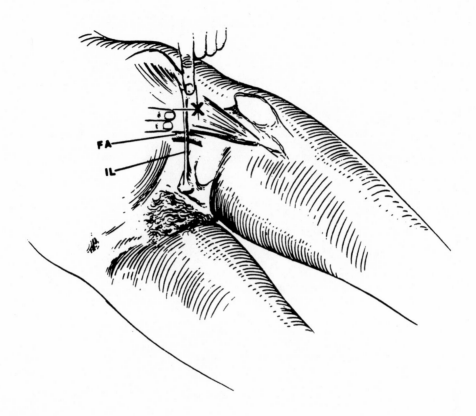

Innervation

Femoral Nerve, Posterior Division Lumbar Plexus, *L2, L3,* L4.

Origin

From the bodies and the transverse processes of the lumbar vertebrae and the iliac fossa.

Insertion

Into the lesser trochanter of the femur.

Position

The patient supine.

187

Electrode Insertion (X)

Two fingerbreadths lateral to the femoral artery (FA) and one fingerbreadth below the inguinal ligament (IL).

Test Maneuver

Patient to flex the thigh with the knee flexed beyond ninety degrees.

Pitfalls

If the electrode is inserted too medially it will contact the neurovascular bundle; if inserted too laterally it will be in the sartorius.

Comment

(a) Involved in lesions of —
   1. High femoral nerve
   2. Posterior Division of the lumbar plexus
   3. L2, L3, L4 roots.
(b) Forms the external portion of the floor of the Scarpa's triangle.

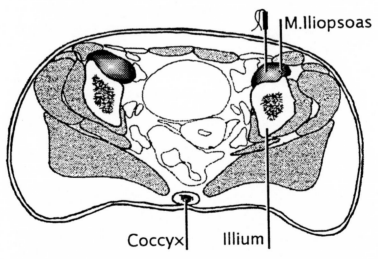

Figure 72. Cross section of the pelvis area just proximal to the hip joint.

PECTINEUS

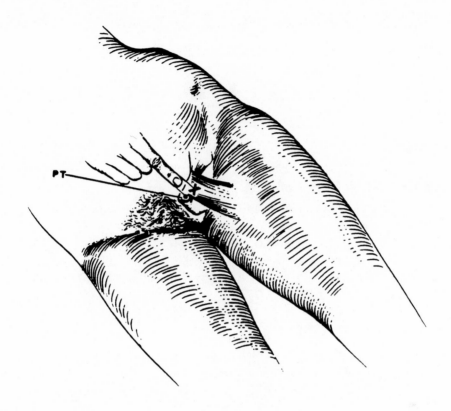

Innervation

Femoral Nerve, Posterior Division Lumbar Plexus, *L2, L3,* L4.

Origin

From the superior ramus of the pubis.

Insertion

Into the upper portion of the pectineal line below the lesser trochanter.

Position

The patient supine.

Electrode Insertion (X)

One fingerbreadth lateral to the pubic tubercle (PT).

Maneuver

Patient to adduct the thigh.

Pitfalls

If the electrode is inserted too medially it will be in the adductor longus; if inserted too laterally it will contact the neurovascular bundle.

Comment

(a) Forms the internal portion of the floor of the Scarpa's triangle.
(b) Involved in lesions of —
    1. Femoral nerve (entrapment) at the inguinal ligament level
    2. Femoral nerve proximal to the inguinal ligaments
    3. Posterior division of the lumbar plexus
    4. L2, L3, L4 roots.

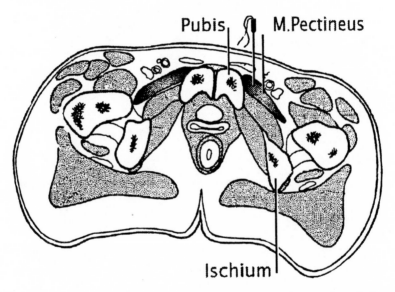

Figure 73. Cross section of the pelvis area through the superior portion of the symphysis pubis.

RECTUS FEMORIS

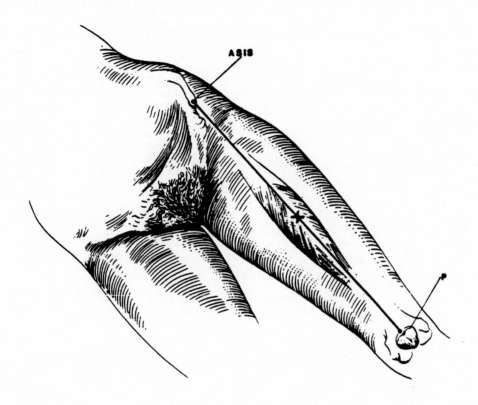

Innervation

Femoral Nerve, Posterior Division Lumbar Plexus, L2, *L3, L4.*

Origin

From the anterior inferior iliac spine and the brim of the acetabulum.

Insertion

Through the patella tendon, on the tibial tubercle.

Position

The patient supine.

Electrode Insertion (X)

On the anterior aspect of the thigh, midway between the superior border of the patella (P) and the anterior superior iliac spine (ASIS).

Test Maneuver

Patient to flex the hip with the knee extended.

Pitfalls

If the electrode is inserted too medially it will be in the vastus intermedius; if inserted too laterally it will be in the vastus lateralis; if inserted too distally and medially it will be in the vastus medialis.

Comment

Involved in lesions of—
1. Femoral nerve (entrapment) at the inguinal ligament level
2. Femoral nerve proximal to the inguinal ligament
3. Posterior division of the lumbar plexus
4. L2, L3, L4.

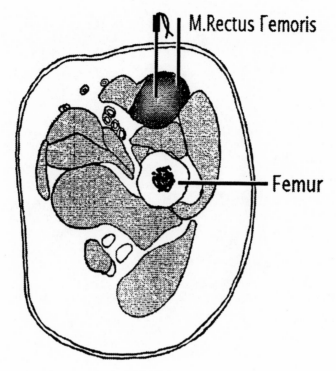

Figure 74. Cross section of the thigh through the junction of the upper and middle third.

SARTORIUS

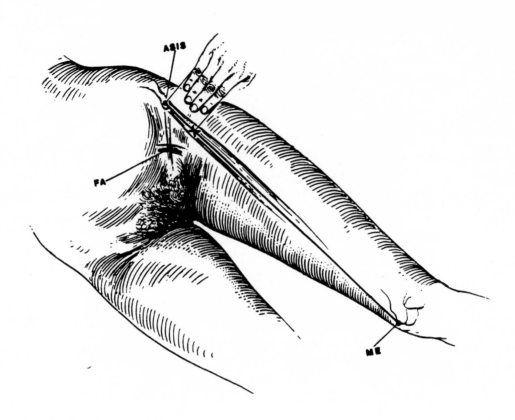

Innervation

Femoral Nerve, Posterior Division Lumbar Plexus, *L2, L3, L4.*

Origin

From the anterior superior iliac spine.

Insertion

Below the medial tibial condyle, on the medial border of the body of the tibia.

Position

The patient supine.

Electrode Insertion (X)

Four fingerbreadths distal to the anterior superior iliac spine (ASIS) along the line to the medial epicondyle (ME) of the tibia. Insert the electrode just lateral to the femoral artery (FA) to a depth of about one-half inch.

Test Maneuver

Patient to flex, abduct and externally rotate thigh.

Pitfalls

If the needle electrode is inserted too deeply or too distally it will be in the rectus femoris; if inserted too medially it will be in the iliacus; if inserted too laterally it will be in the tensor fascia lata.

Comment

Involved in lesions of —
1. Femoral nerve (entrapment) at the inguinal ligament level
2. Femoral nerve proximal to the inguinal ligament
3. Posterior division of the lumbar plexus
4. L2, L3, L4.

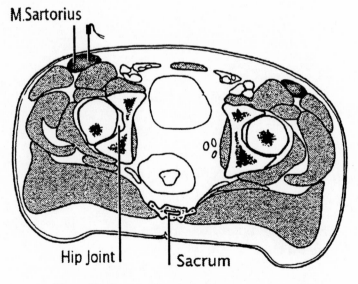

Figure 75. Cross section through the hip joint.

SEMIMEMBRANOSUS

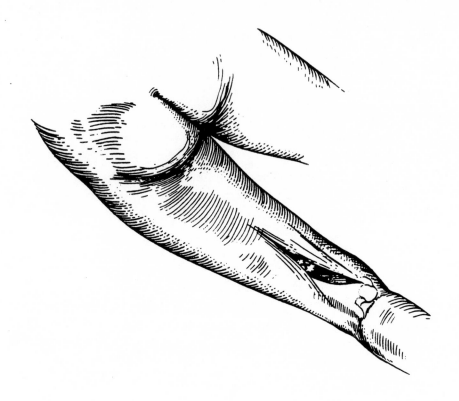

Innervation

Sciatic Nerve (Tibial Portion), Anterior Division Sacral Plexus, L5, S1, S2.

Origin

From the ischial tuberosity.

Insertion

On the medial condyle of the tibia and through a fibrous expansion into the lateral femoral condyle.

Position

The patient prone.

Electrode Insertion (X)

Insert the electrode laterally to the semitendinosus tendon in the apex of the "V" between the semitendinosus tendon and the biceps femoris.

Test Maneuver

Patient to flex the knee and internally rotate the tibia.

Pitfalls

If the electrode is inserted too medially it will be in the semitendinosus; if inserted too laterally it will be the short head of the biceps or into the sciatic nerve; if inserted too deeply it will be in the adductor magnus.

Comment

Involved in lesions of—
1. Sciatic nerve
2. Anterior division of the sacral plexus
3. L5, S1, S2.

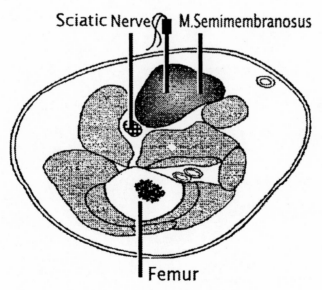

Figure 76. Cross section of the thigh through the lower third.

SEMITENDINOSUS

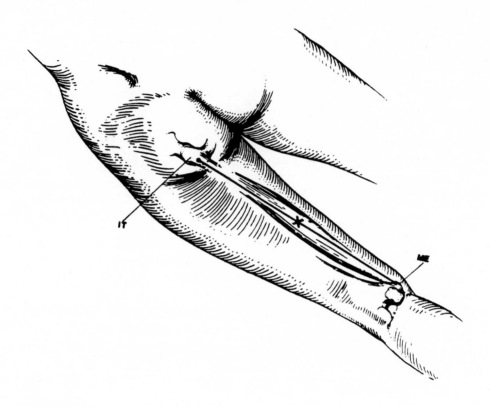

Innervation

Sciatic Nerve (Tibial Portion), Anterior Division Sacral Plexus, L5, S1, S2.

Origin

From the ischial tuberosity.

Insertion

On the medial condyle of the tibia.

Position

The patient prone.

Electrode Insertion (X)

Midway on a line between the medial epicondyle (ME) of the femur and the ischial tuberosity (IT).

Test Maneuver

Patient to flex the knee and internally rotate the tibia;

Pitfalls

If the electrode is inserted too laterally it will be in the long head of the biceps; if inserted too medially or too deeply it will be in the semimembranosus.

Comment

Involved in lesions of —
1. Sciatic nerve
2. Anterior division sacral plexus
3. L5, S1, S2 roots.

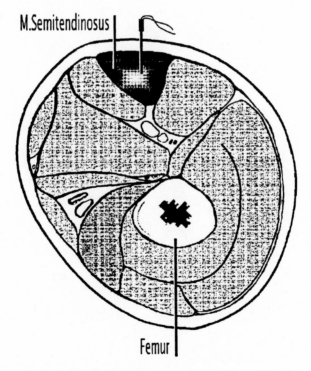

Figure 77. Cross section of the thigh through the midportion.

TENSOR FASCIE LATAE

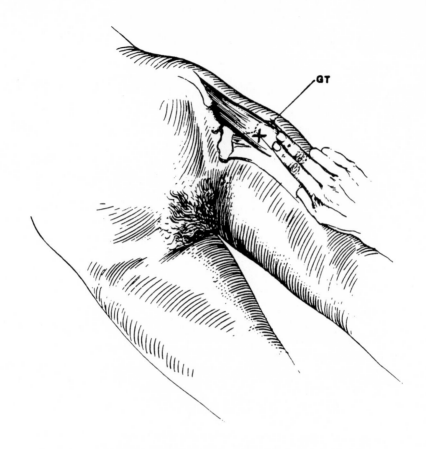

Innervation

Superior Gluteal Nerve, Sacral Plexus, L4, *L5, S1.*

Origin

From outer lip of the anterior portion of iliac crest of the ilium.

Insertion

On the iliotibial tract, just below the greater trochanter.

Position

The patient supine.

Electrode Insertion (X)

Two fingerbreadths anterior to the greater trochanter (GT).

Test Maneuver

Patient to abduct thigh with hip flexed.

Pitfalls

If the electrode is inserted too anteriorly it will be in the sartorius or rectus femoris; if inserted too deeply it will be in the vastus lateralis; if inserted too posteriorly it will be in the gluteus medius.

Comment

Involved in lesions of—
1. Superior gluteal nerve
2. Posterior division of the sacral plexus
3. L4, L5, S1 roots.

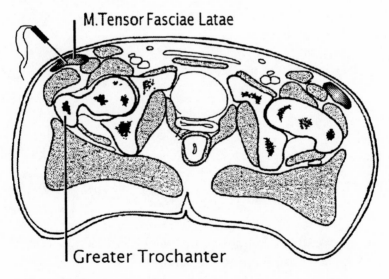

Figure 78. Cross section of the pelvis through the greater trochanter.

VASTUS INTERMEDIUS

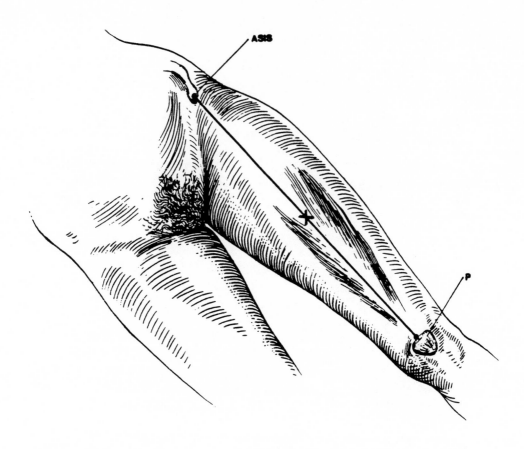

Innervation

Femoral Nerve, Posterior Division Lumbar Plexus, *L2, L3, L4.*

Origin

From the upper three-fourths of the shaft of the femur and from the anterior surface as high as the introchanteric line.

Insertion

Through the quadriceps tendon onto the tibial tubercle.

Position

The patient supine.

Electrode Insertion

Midway between the superior border of the patella (P) and the anterior superior iliac spine (ASIS). The electrode is inserted to the bone and withdrawn slightly.

Test Maneuver

Patient to lift heel from plinth with knee extended.

Pitfalls

If the electrode is inserted too superficially it will be in the rectus femoris; if inserted too laterally it will be in the vastus lateralis; if inserted too medially it will be in the vastus medialis or sartorius.

Comment

Involved in lesions of —
1. Femoral nerve (entrapment) at the inguinal ligament level
2. Femoral nerve proximal to the inguinal ligament
3. Posterior division of the lumbar plexus
4. L2, L3, L4 roots.

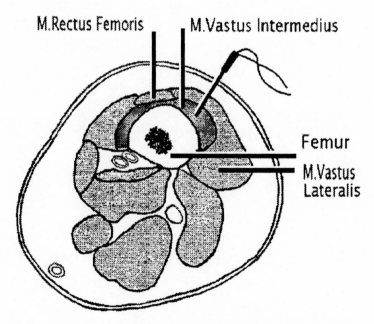

Figure 79. Cross section of the thigh through the middle and distal third.

VASTUS LATERALIS

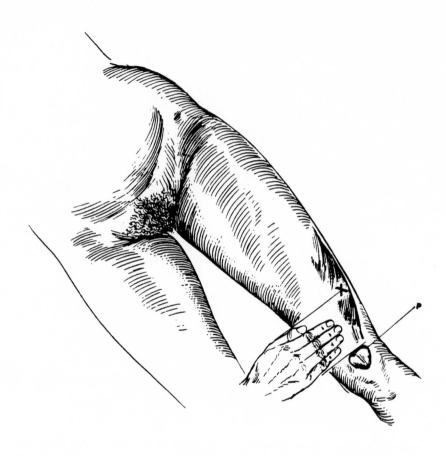

Innervation

Femoral Nerve, Posterior Division Lumbar Plexus, L2, *L3, L4.*

Origin

From the intertrochanteric line, the linea aspera and the medial sypracondylar line.

Insertion

Through the quadriceps tendon onto the tibial tubercle.

Position

The patient supine.

Electrode Insertion (X)

Over the lateral aspect of the thigh, one handbreadth above the patella (P).

Test Maneuver

Patient to lift heel from plinth with knee extended.

Pitfalls

If the electrode is inserted too posteriorly it will be in the biceps femoris; if inserted too medially it will be in the rectus femoris.

Comment

Involved in lesions of —
1. Femoral nerve (entrapment) at the inguinal ligament level
2. Femoral nerve proximal to the inguinal ligament
3. Posterior division of the lumbar plexus
4. L2, L3, L4 roots.

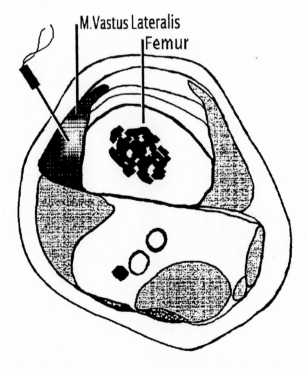

Figure 80. Cross section of the thigh just proximal to the patella.

VASTUS MEDIALIS

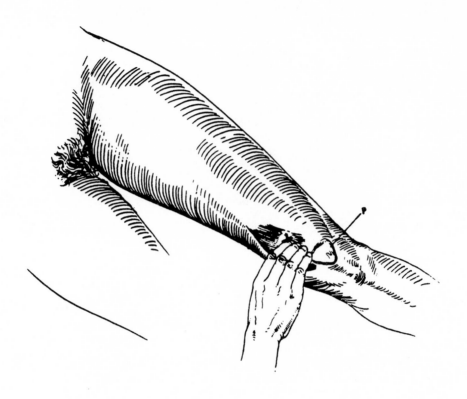

Innervation

Femoral Nerve, Posterior Division Lumbar Plexus, L2, *L3, L4.*

Origin

From the medial lip of the linea aspera and upper part of the supracondylar line.

Insertion

Through the quadriceps tendon onto the tibial tubercle.

Position

The patient supine.

Electrode Insertion (X)

Four fingerbreadths proximal to the superiomedial angle of the patella (P).

Test Maneuver

Patient to lift heel from plinth with knee extended.

Pitfalls

If the electrode is inserted too posteriorly it will be in the sartorius or gracilis; if inserted too anteriorly it will be in the rectus femoris.

Comment

(a) Used as recording muscle for femoral nerve motor conduction study
(b) Involved in lesions of —
   1. Femoral nerve (entrapment) at the inguinal ligaments
   2. Intrapelvic femoral nerve
   3. Posterior division of lumbar plexus
   4. L2, L3, L4 nerve roots.

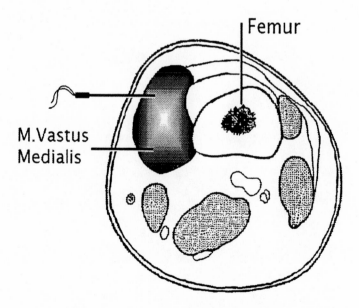

Figure 81. Cross section of the thigh through the distal third.

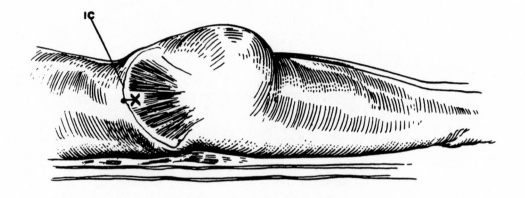

SECTION IX
PELVIS AND HIP JOINT

GLUTEUS MAXIMUS

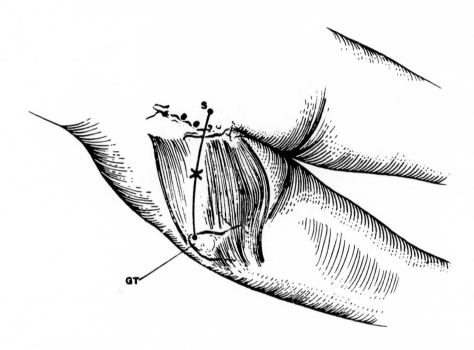

Innervation

Inferior Gluteal Nerve, Sacral Plexus, L5, *S1, S2.*

Origin

From the gluteal line, the posterior surface of the sacrum and coccyx, and the sacrotuberous ligament.

Insertion

Into the iliotibial tract, the gluteal ridge, and the linea aspera of the femur.

Position

The patient prone.

Electrode Insertion (X)

The electrode is inserted to a depth of one to three inches midway between the greater trochanter (GT) and the sacrum (S).

Test Maneuver

Patient to extend the hip with the knee flexed.

Pitfalls

None.

Comment

(a) Involved in lesions of —
1. Inferior gluteal nerve
2. Posterior division of sacral plexus
3. L5, S1, S2 nerve roots.
(b) A frequent site of intramuscular injection therefore, pathological findings may be misleading.

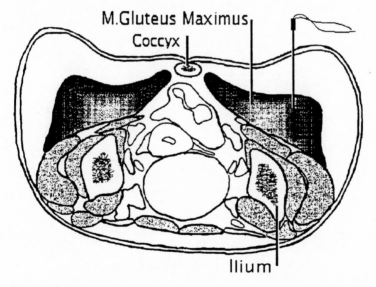

Figure 82. Cross section of the pelvis area just proximal to the hip joint.

GLUTEUS MEDIUS

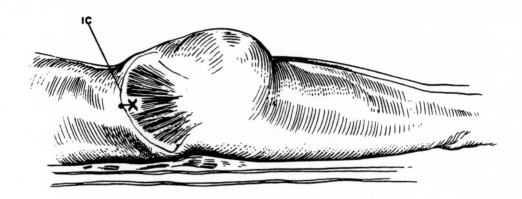

Innervation

Superior Gluteal Nerve, L4, L5, S1.

Origin

From the anterior gluteal line and the crest of the ilium.

Insertion

Into the greater trochanter.

Position

The patient prone.

Electrode Insertion (X)

One inch distal to the midpoint of the iliac crest (IC).

Test Maneuver

Patient to abduct the thigh.

Pitfalls

If the electrode is inserted too posteriorly it will be in the gluteus maximus; if inserted too anteriorly it will be in the tensa fascia lata; if inserted too distally it will be in either the gluteus minimus or maximus.

212

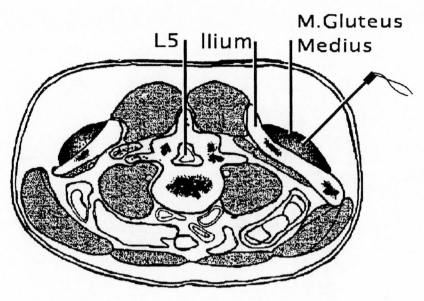

Figure 83. Cross section of the pelvis through the L5 level.

GLUTEUS MINIMUS

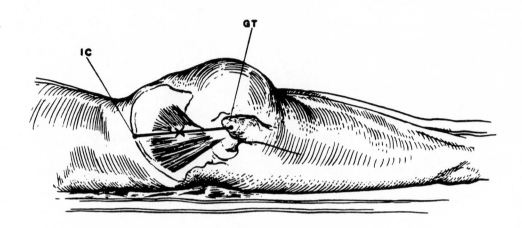

Innervation

Superior Gluteal Nerve, Sacral Plexus, L4, *L5*, S1.

Origin

From the lateral surface of the ilium, between the anterior and inferior gluteal line.

Insertion

Into the anterior surface of the greater trochanter.

Position

The patient prone.

Electrode Insertion (X)

Insert electrode midway between midpoint of the iliac crest (IC) and greater trochanter (GT) deep to bone and withdraw slightly.

Test Maneuver

Patient to abduct the thigh.

Pitfalls

If the electrode is inserted too superficially it will be in the gluteus medius.

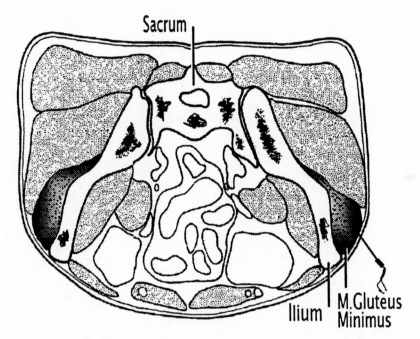

Figure 84. Cross section of the pelvis through the middle of the sacral mass.

OBTURATOR INTERNUS AND GEMELLI*

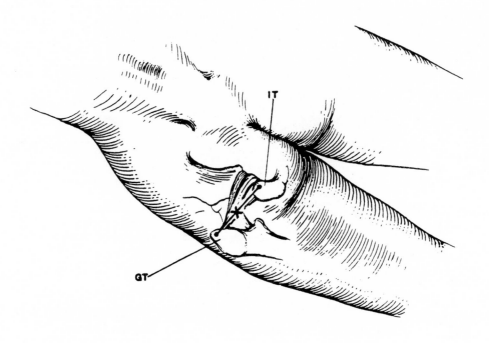

Innervation

Obturator Internus and Superior Gemellus: Obturator Internus Nerve, Sacral Plexus, L5, *S1, S2.*

Inferior Gemellus: Quadratus Femoris Nerve, Sacral Plexus L4, *L5,* S1, S2.

Both Nerves: Arise From the Proximal Segment of the Tibial Portion of the Sciatic Nerve.

Origin

From the ischial spine, the ischial tuberosity, the obturator membrane and the adjacent bone.

Insertion

Into the medial side of the greater trochanter.

---

*The gemelli are considered the extra pelvic portion of the obturator internus.

216

Position

The patient prone.

Electrode Insertion

Insert electrode to bone and withdraw slightly at a point midway between the ischial tuberosity (IT) and the posterosuperior aspect of greater trochanter (GT). The electrode will travel through the gluteus maximus muscle.

Test Maneuver

Patient to externally rotate the thigh with the leg extended.

Pitfalls

If the electrode is inserted too medially it will contact the sciatic nerve; if inserted too superficially it will be in the gluteus maximus; if inserted too distally it will be in the quadratus femoris; if inserted too proximally it will be in the piriformis.

Comment

Involved in lesions of the lumbosacral plexus close to the spine or in L5, S1, S2 radiculopathies.

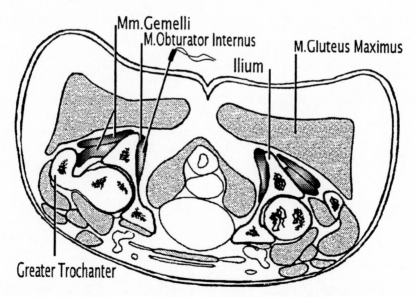

Figure 85. Cross section of the pelvis through the midportion of the hip joint.

PIRIFORMIS

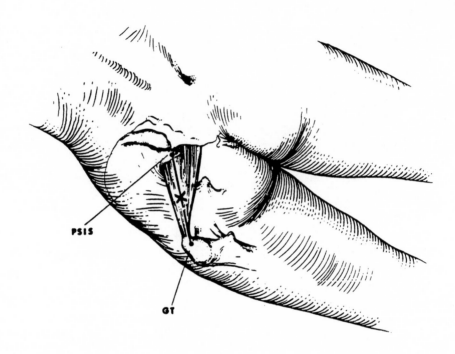

Innervation

Nerve to the Piriformis S1, S2.

Origin

From the front of the sacrum.

Insertion

Into the piriform fossa of the greater trochanter.

Position

The patient prone.

Electrode Insertion (X)

Insert the electrode deep to bone at the midpoint of a line between the posterior inferior iliac spine (SIS) and the posterior-superior margin of the greater trochanter (GT), then withdraw slightly. The electrode will travel through the gluteus maximus muscle.

Test Maneuver

Patient to externally rotate thigh.

Pitfalls

If the electrode is inserted too superficially it will be in the gluteus maximus; if inserted too caudally it will be on the obturator internus or gemelli.

Comment

(a) The sciatic nerve may be entrapped as it crosses this muscle (piriformis syndrome).
(b) Involved in lesions of S1 and S2. This muscle is innervated directly from these roots.

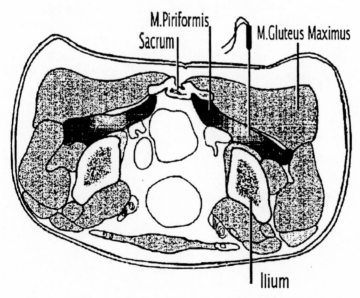

Figure 86. Cross section of the pelvis at the lower sacral mass.

QUADRATUS FEMORIS

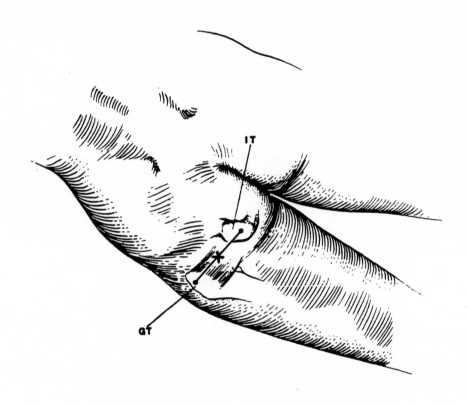

Innervation

Nerve to the Quadratus Femoris, Sciatic Nerve (Tibial Portion), L4, L5, S1.

Origin

From the ischial tuberosity deep to the hamstrings.

Insertion

Into the quadrate tubercle of the femur.

Position

The patient prone.

Electrode Insertion (X)

Midway between the greater trochanter (GT) and the ischial tuberosity (IT). The electrode should contact bone and then be withdrawn slightly. The electrode will travel through the gluteus maximus muscle.

Test Maneuver

Patient to externally rotate thigh.

Pitfalls

If the electrode is inserted too superficially it will be in the gluteus maximus or medius; if inserted too distally it will be in the hamstring group.

Comment

Involved in lesions of sciatic nerve at its junction with the sacral plexus or L4, L5, S1 roots.

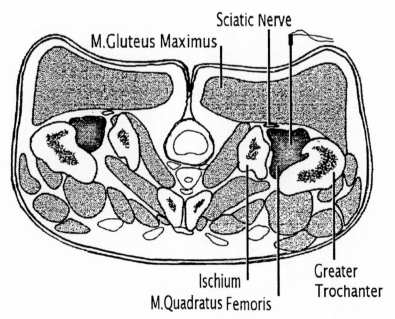

Figure 87. Cross section of the pelvis through the inferior portion of the sumphisis pubis.

THE TRUNK

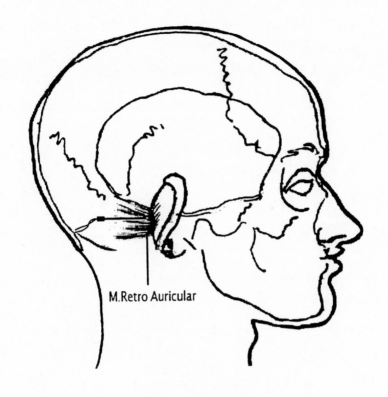

M.Retro Auricular

SECTION X
MUSCLES INNERVATED BY CRANIAL NERVES

FACIAL NERVE (NUMBER 7)

FACIAL (VII)

The facial nerve provides the motor innervation of all the muscles in the face (muscles of expression) and it divides into 7 branches after exiting from the stylomastoid foramen. These branches are:

(a) *Post Auricular Nerve:* Supplies the *retroauricular muscle* and the occipital belly of the occipitofrontalis muscle (This branch leaves the main trunk of the facial nerve before the nerve enters the postero-medial aspect of the parotid gland).

The terminal branches of the facial nerve are subject to great variation, and the following description may occur in a certain percentage of the cases.

(b) *Temporal Branches:* Supplies the *orbicularis oculi* and the frontal portion of *occipitofrontalis.*

(c) *Mandibular Branch:* Supplies the depressor anguli oris and muscles of the chin.

(d) *Cervical Branch:* Supplies the platysma.

(e) *Zygomatic Branches:* Supplies the zygomatic muscle and *orbicularis oculi.*

(f) *Superficial Buccal Branches:* Supplies the *orbicularis oris.*

(g) *Deep Buccal Branch:* Supplies the buccinator and the muscles of the nose.

Only the following muscles will be described as they are the most commonly investigated:

Retroauricular
Frontalis
Orbicularis oculi
Elevator nostril
Orbicularis oris

RETRO AURICULAR OR
AURICULARIS POSTERIOR

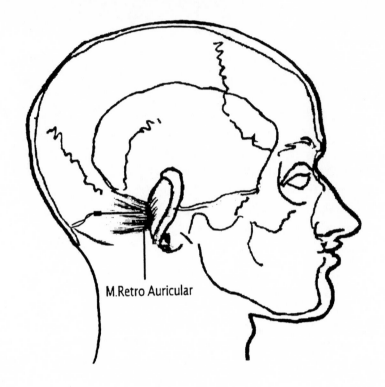

M.Retro Auricular

Origin

From the mastoid part of the temporal bone.

Insertion

To the cranial aspect of the auricle.

Position

Patient in supine position with head rotated to the side not under study.

Electrode Insertion

The auricle is pulled forward and several small creases will appear at the angle formed between the auricle and the scalp. These creases represent the stretching of the muscle underneath. The electrode is placed at that point to ¼ to ½ inch in depth.

Test Maneuver

The patient is asked to wiggle his ear. Even though the actual motion of the auricle may not be seen, however, electrical activity is generally seen.

Pitfalls

None.

Comments

(1) The study of this muscle could help in localizing facial nerve lesion occurring in the parotid gland. In this case, the muscle will show normal electrical activity.

(2) This muscle is involved in lesions of the facial nerve occurring at the motor nucleus of the 7th C.N., down to the stylomastoid foramen.

ORBICULARIS OCULI

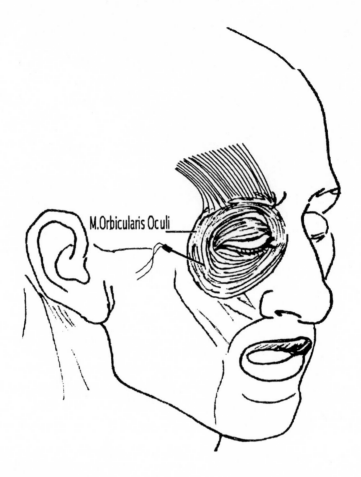

M.Orbicularis Oculi

Origin and Insertion

Two Parts: The central, which travels within the eyelids, and the orbital, which is larger and thicker, encircle the central and insert in the medial palpebral ligament, the bone above and below the ligament, spread around the eyebrows, the temporal region and the cheek.

Position

The patient is supine with the head in neutral position.

Electrode Insertion

Palpate the lateral portion of the eye fossa (bone) and direct the tip of the electrode at a 25–30 angle with the skin, in a medial and downward direction. It will penetrate the lower lip portion of the orbicularis oculi. .

230

Test Maneuver

Ask the patient to wink or blink very gently. This maneuver should not be repeated too often because the motion of the electrode can produce some soft tissue damage which may lead to swelling and/or hemorrhage (black eye) due to the extreme looseness of the tissues in the infraorbital area.

Pitfalls

If the electrode is inserted too perpendicular to the skin, it may enter the orbit which can damage the eyeball.

Comments

(1) This muscle is used as a pick-up muscle for the blink reflex test.
(2) This muscle is involved in all nuclear and infranuclear lesions of the facial nerve.

DILATOR NARIS

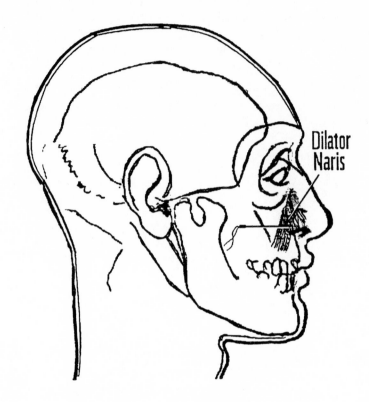

Dilator
Naris

Origin

From the front of the maxilla above the incisor and canine teeth.

Insertion

Into the ALA of the nostril.

Position

Patient is supine with head in neutral position.

Electrode Insertion

Because of the small size of the muscle, needle electrode is very seldom used. Instead, a surface electrode (8mm DISC) is placed over the skin covering the muscle. This muscle is used as the reference electrode during the blink reflex.

Test Maneuver

Ask patient to take a deep breath through the nose.

Pitfalls

None.

Comments

(1) This muscle is involved in all types of facial nerve lesions.
(2) The action of this muscle becomes evident during laborious breathing.

ORBICULARIS ORIS

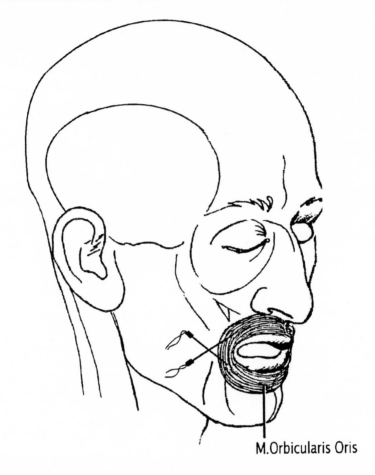

M.Orbicularis Oris

As a sphincter muscle around the mouth, this muscle is anchored to the nasal septum and the maxilla above and the mandible below. There is no clear point of origin or insertion. This muscle is in close connection with several small muscles, which give an infinite variety of expressions to the facial activity.

Position

Patient is supine with head in neutral position.

Electrode Insertion

One-finger's breadth lateral to the angle of the mouth the electrode is inserted through the skin at a 20 angle and is advanced toward either the upper or the lower lip. The tip of the electrode should not be closer than 2cm from the midline.

Test Maneuver

The patient is asked to pucker his lips.

Pitfalls

(1) If the electrode is inserted too vertically to the skin, the tip may end up in the oral cavity.
(2) If the tip of the electrode is too close to the midline, it can pick-up electrical activity from the opposite half of the muscle due to cross over innervation.

Comments

One of the important functions of this muscle is to open and close the mouth voluntarily for a variety of reasons. Furthermore, in conjunction with all of the small muscles it is attached to, it becomes an important muscle that conveys a large number of different emotional states associated with mirth or grief; delight or sadness; fear or despair. The paralysis of part of this sphincter, produces a marked impact on the ability to express all of these emotional states.

OCCIPITOFRONTALIS

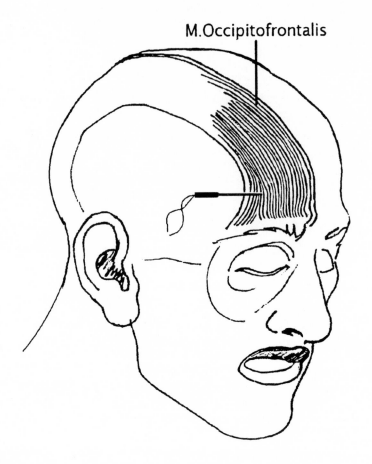

M.Occipitofrontalis

Origin

From the epicranial aponeurosis at the level of the coronal suture in both sides.

Insertion

It descends over the frontal bone to the edge of the orbital margin where it interlaces with the fibers of the orbicularis oculi without having any bone attachment.

Position

The patient is in supine position with the muscle under study closer to the examiner.

Electrode Insertion

One-finger's breadth superior to the orbital margin and two-fingers' breadth from the midline.

Test Maneuver

The patient is asked to raise his eyebrows (furrow the forehead transversely).

Pitfalls

(1) If the electrode is inserted too low, it may enter the orbicularis oculi.

(2) If inserted too close to the midline, electrical activity may be found which may be coming from the opposite side due to some crossover innervation of the muscle. It is recommended that the electrode be inserted in a way that the tip will be away from the midline.

Comments

(1) This muscle is involved in all nuclear and infranuclear lesions of the facial nerve (bell's palsy; cerebellar-pontine angle tumor; fracture of the petrous part of the temporal bone; parotid gland tumors).

HYPOGLOSSAL NERVE (NUMBER 12)

TONGUE

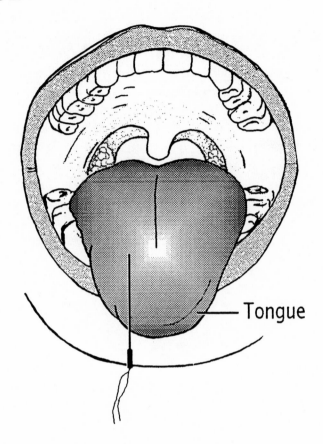

Tongue

Innervation

Cranial Nerve #12 Hypoglossal

Origin

(a) Genioglossus: From the genial tuberosity of the mandible.
(b) Hypoglossus: From the body and greater horn of the hyoid bone.
(c) Styloglossus: From the front tip of the styloid process and the stylohyoid ligament.

Insertion

The three paired muscles converge to join in a latticework with the intrinsic tongue muscle.

Position

Patient in sitting position.

239

Electrode Insertion

The patient is asked to stick out his tongue. The examiner holds the tongue with a gauze and keeps it steady. With the other hand, the electrode (coaxial, disposable, 25mm in length) is inserted on one side of the tongue. The patient is now asked to pull his tongue back into the mouth and is asked to close his mouth and relax. When relaxation is obtained, the back ground electrical activity of the tongue will cease. If fibrillations and/or fasciculations are present, they can be seen at this time. To assess the muscle activity at maximal effort, the patient is asked to open his mouth and stick out his tongue. It should be remembered that the tongue is a muscle that pushes rather than pulls. Therefore, when the tongue protrudes from the mouth, it is actually producing a contraction.

Test Maneuver

Stick tongue out of the mouth.

Pitfalls

None.

Comments

The tongue electromyography is usually done in patients suspected of suffering from A.L.S. This study requires a great deal of patient's cooperation. The entire procedure should be fully explained to the patient before it starts.
The tongue is a muscle that is very difficult to bring to full relaxation. Therefore the technique should be followed meticulously. When the tongue presents unequal strength on both sides, the tip deviates toward the weak side when protruded. The weak half becomes atrophied and exhibits deep furrows.

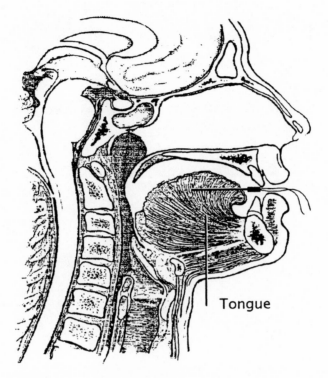

Figure 88. The tongue is resting; no electrical activity should be present.

SPINAL ACCESSORY (NUMBER 11)

STERNO–CLEIDO–MASTOID (S.C.M.)

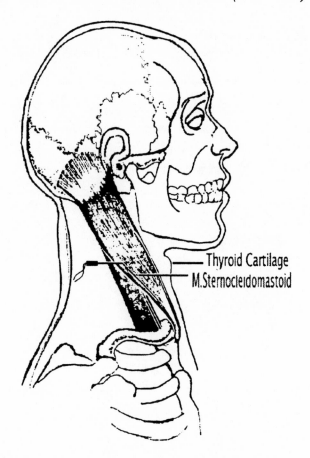

Thyroid Cartilage
M.Sternocleidomastoid

Innervation

By the spinal accessory nerve which is formed by the spinal roots (upper 5 cervical ventral roots); they ascend through the foramen magnus, to exit through the jugular foramen, after joining the cranial roots.

Origin

Two heads: (a) Sternal or medial from the anterior surface of the manubrium sterni, (b) Clavicular or lateral from the upper surface of the medial third of the clavicle.

Insertion

The two heads merge together and the muscle end over the mastoid process. Before the muscle end, it is pierced by the spinal accessory nerve.

Position

The patient is in supine position with the head in neutral position.

Electrode Insertion

Four-fingers' breadth cephalad to the muscle origin (at the level of the thyroid cartilage) (Adam's apple). Because of the muscle's mobility and the skin looseness, it is practical to pinch the muscle between the index and thumb to anchor it firmly and to allow a safer electrode insertion.

Test Maneuver

The patient is asked to either flex the head or to perform a combined motion of slight head extension and rotation to the opposite side that is being tested (to bring the mastoid process closer to the manubrium sterni).

Pitfalls

1. Too deep: The electrode might puncture the carotid artery or the jugular vein.
2. Too posterior and too deep: The electrode might damage part of the brachial plexus.
3. Too low and too deep: The electrode might puncture the dome of the lung.

Comments

1. The S.C.M. constitute the boundary between the anterior and posterior triangle of the neck.
2. Contrary to the trapezius, the S.C.M. is not involved when the spinal accessory nerve is damaged during supraclavicular lymph node biopsy.
3. It might become an important accessory breathing muscle.
4. This muscle is often involved in torticollis or dystonia musculorum.

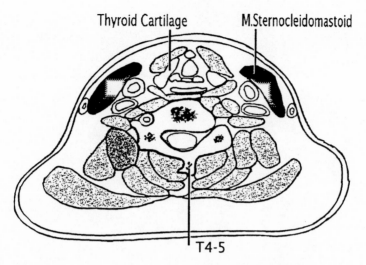

Figure 89. Cross section at the T4-5 vertebral level (thyroid cartilage level).

TRAPEZIUS, LOWER

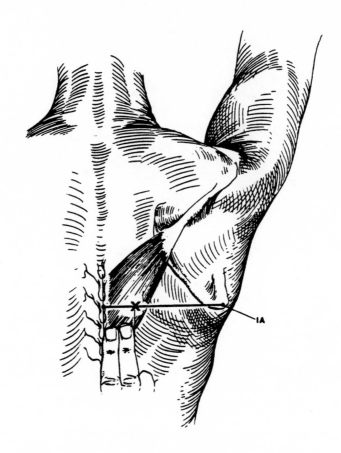

Innervation

Spinal Portion of Accessory Nerve and Twigs from C3, C4.

Origin

Spinous processes of lower thoracic vertebrae.

Insertion

The spine of the scapula.

Position

Patient prone with arm extended overhead.

246

Electrode Insertion (X)

On a line perpendicular to the vertebral column at the level of the inferior angle (IA) of the scapula, two fingerbreadths from the spinous process of that vertebra.

Test Maneuver

Elevate arm from plinth.

Pitfalls

If needle electrode is inserted too deeply or too caudally it will be in the latissimus dorsi.

Comment

This muscle may be involved due to injury to its innervation in cervical lymph node biopsy.

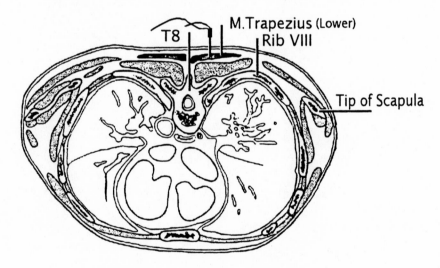

Figure 90. Cross section at the T8 level.

TRAPEZIUS, MIDDLE

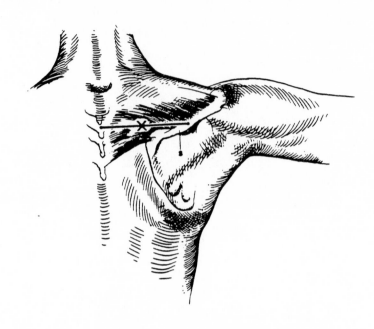

Innervation

Spinal Portion of Accessory Nerve and Twigs From C3 and C4.

Origin

The seventh cervical and spinous processes of upper thoracic vertebrae.

Insertion

The acromion process and spine of scapula.

Position

The patient prone with arm abducted to ninety degrees and elbow flexed over the edge of plinth.

Electrode Insertion (X)

Midway between the midpoint of spine (S) of scapula and spinous process of vertebra at the same level.

Test Maneuver

Adduct scapula by elevation of arm from plinth.

Pitfalls

If needle electrode is inserted too deeply it will be in the rhomboideus.

Comment

This muscle may be involved due to injury to its innervation in cervical lymph node biopsy.

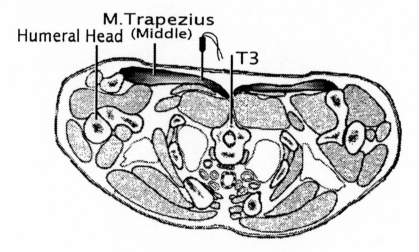

Figure 91. Cross section at the T3 level.

TRAPEZIUS, UPPER

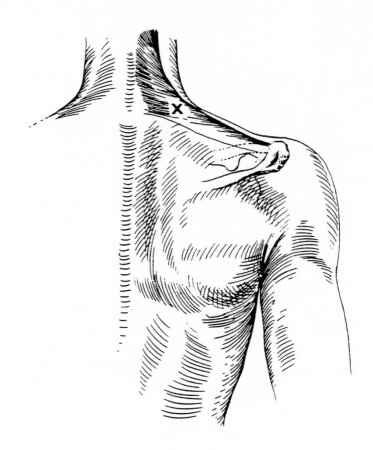

Innervation

Spinal Portion of Accessory Nerve and Twigs from C3 and C4.

Origin

Occipital bone and ligamentum nuchae.

Insertion

The outer third of clavicle.

Position

The patient prone.

Electrode Insertion (X)

At angle of neck and shoulder.

Test Maneuver

Shrug shoulder.

Pitfalls

If needle electrode is inserted too deeply it will be in the levator scapula.

Comment

This muscle may be involved due to injury to its innervation in cervical lymph node biopsy.

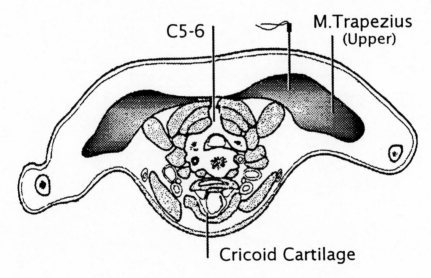

Figure 92. Cross section at the C5–6 level.

TRIGEMINAL NERVE (NUMBER 5)

A. TEMPORAL MUSCLE

M. Temporalis

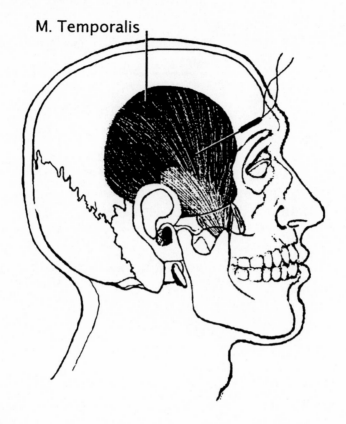

Innervation

By the deep temporal nerve, which branches off the anterior trunk of the mandibular nerve (3rd division of the trigeminal nerve).

Origin

From the floor of temporal fossa as well as the fascia covering the muscle.

Insertion

Into the apex and the anterior border of the coronoid process of the mandible.

Position

The patient is either seated with the head resting on a headrest or lying supine with the head in neutral position.

Electrode Insertion

Two-fingers' breadth above the zygomatic arch, and two-fingers' breadth posterior to the eye commissurae.

Test Maneuver

The patient is asked to clench his teeth.

Pitfalls

If inserted too close to the external eye orbit, it could be in the orbicularis oculi. If inserted too close to the zygomatic arch, it could be in the tendinous portion of the temporal muscle.

Comments

(a) This muscle could be involved in trigeminal neuritis.
(b) Caution should be exercised to avoid piercing the temporal artery.

B. MASSETER MUSCLE

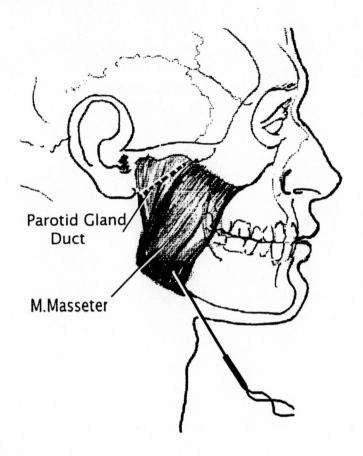

Parotid Gland
Duct

M.Masseter

Innervation

Nerve to the masseter which branches off the anterior trunk of the mandibular nerve.

Origin

From the zygomatic arch, lower border.

Insertion

The muscular and tendinous part into the lateral aspect of the coronoid process of the mandible.

Position

Patient is either seated with the head resting on a headrest or lying supine with the head in neutral position.

Electrode Insertion

One-finger's breadth posterior to the anterior edge of the muscle (recognizable when patient clenches his teeth or palpating the facial artery which winds around the anterior edge of the muscle) and one-finger's breadth cephalad to the lower edge of the mandible.

Test Maneuver

The patient is asked to clench his teeth.

Pitfalls

If electrode is inserted too close to the zygomatic arch, the duct of the parotid gland can be damaged.
If electrode is inserted close to the posterior edge of the muscle, it will go through the parotid gland.
If electrode is inserted too close to the anterior edge of the muscle, the tip may end up in the mouth.

Comments

(a) This muscle could be involved in trigeminal neuritis.
(b) The parotid gland and/or the parotid duct can be compromised.
(c) The muscle can be damaged during dissection for parotid gland tumors.

VAGUS NERVE (NUMBER 10)

CRICOTHYROID

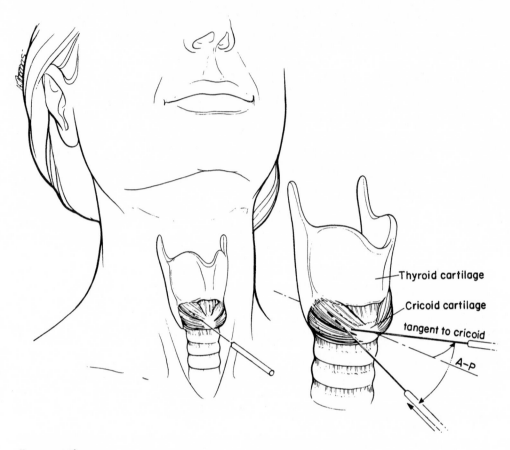

Thyroid cartilage

Cricoid cartilage

tangent to cricoid

A~P

Innervation

External branch of the superior laryngeal nerve which branches off the middle of the inferior ganglion of the vagus nerve.

Origin

Antero-lateral surface of the cricoid cartilage (arch).

Insertion

Inferior border of the thyroid lamina and anterior aspect of the inferior thyroid horn.

Position

The patient is supine with the head in neutral position. A pillow is placed across the shoulders to allow the head to be slightly hyper-extended. The skin covering the space between the cricoid and the thyroid cartilage is infiltrated with 1% xilocaine intracutaneously (to produce "orange skin"). This infiltration is done 1cm from the midline bilaterally. When introducing the electrode, the larynx should be steady.

Electrode Insertion

A 25mm coaxial disposable EMG electromyography electrode is inserted through the anesthetized skin tangential to the upper border of the cricoid arch in a superior and lateral direction. During the advancement of the electrode the patient vocalizes the vowel "e." Much higher electrical activity is found when the vocalization of "e" is done at a high pitch rather than at a low pitch.

Test Maneuver

The electrical output of the muscle increases greatly when the high pitched noise is performed. When the patient is asked to elevate his head from the table, only distant electrical activity should be seen (strap muscles distant activity).

Pitfalls

(1) If the electrode is too superficial, it will be in the sternohyoid muscle. If it is too deep it will be in the lateral cricoarytenoid muscle.*

(2) If this nerve is affected at the same time as the recurrent laryngeal, the problem is affecting the vagus nerve or vagus nucleus. There will be alteration of the vocal cord function and position.

(3) In isolated lesions of this nerve, the patient will have difficulty attaining high voice tones.

---

*Minoru Hirand et al: Use of hookwire electrodes for electromyography of the intrinsic laryngeal muscles. Journal of Speech and Hearing Research 12; 362–373, 1969.

VOCALIS OR THYROARYTENOID MUSCLE

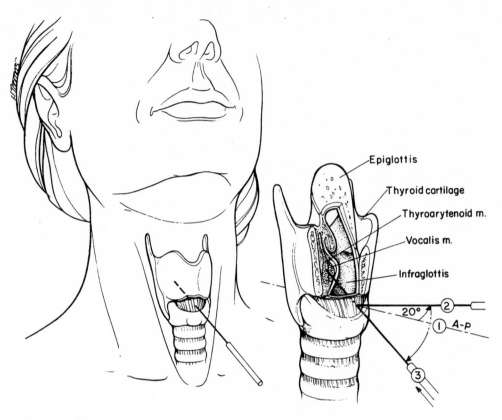

Epiglottis

Thyroid cartilage

Thyroarytenoid m.

Vocalis m.

Infraglottis

20°

A-P

Innervation

Recurrent laryngeal nerve from the vagus nerve.

Origin

From the posterior aspect of the thyroid cartilage.

Insertion

To the postero-lateral border and muscular process of the arytenoid cartilage.

Position

The patient is supine with the head in neutral position. A pillow is placed across the shoulders to allow the head to be slightly hyper-extended. This facilitates the recognition of the thyroid and the cri-coid cartilages. The skin covering the space between the thyroid and the cricoid cartilage is anesthetized with 1% xilocaine. This permits the patient to feel less pain which in turn decreases the tension in the patient and the tendency to evoke the swallowing reflex. For purposes of introducing the electrode, the patient's larynx should be steady.

Electrode Insertion

A 50mm coaxial disposable EMG electrode is inserted through the skin and the cricothyroid membrane. As soon as the electrode pierces the membrane, its direction is oriented to about 20° laterally and 45° superiorly or proximally. The intention is to advance the electrode submucosaly, avoiding entering the subglottic cavity.* Other investigators using the same entrance, prefer to enter the subglottic cavity and then angle the electrode cephalad and to the side of the muscle that is to be studied.† With either technique, it is advisable to advance the electrode while the patient is phonating. The electrical activity increases as the electrode approaches the muscle.

Test Maneuver

The electrical activity increases during glottal stop (valsalva); waxes and wanes with breathing activity (inspiration = increase; expiration = decrease); vocalizing ('e').

Pitfalls

If the electrode's tip is in the subglottic cavity, the electromyographic machine produces a large amount of interference noise. If the electrode is too deep, it may reach the lateral cricoarytenoid muscle.

Comments

(1) The thyroid and cricoid cartilages are much more developed in males than in females. Therefore, the identification of the anatomic landmarks is much easier and the procedure simpler in males than in females.

(2) The recurrent laryngeal nerve on the right side can be affected in patients with aneurism of the aortic arch; both nerves can be

---

*Blair, R et al.: Laryngeal electromyography: Technique and application. Otolaryngology Clin. North Amer. 1978; 11:225.

†Minoru Hirand et al.: Use of hook-wire electrodes for electromyography of the intrinsic laryngeal muscles. Journal of Speech and Hearing Research 12; 362–373, 1969.

damaged in tumors invading the mediastinum; in vagal neuritis; in lesions of the nucleus of the vagal nerve (A.L.S.).

(3) The recurrent laryngeal nerve innervates all the intrinsic laryngeal muscles except the cricothyroid (superior laryngeal nerve).

SECTION XI
MUSCLES OF
THE PERINEAL REGION

PELVIC DIAPHRAGM

A. SPHINCTER ANI EXTERNUS (RECTAL SPHINCTER)

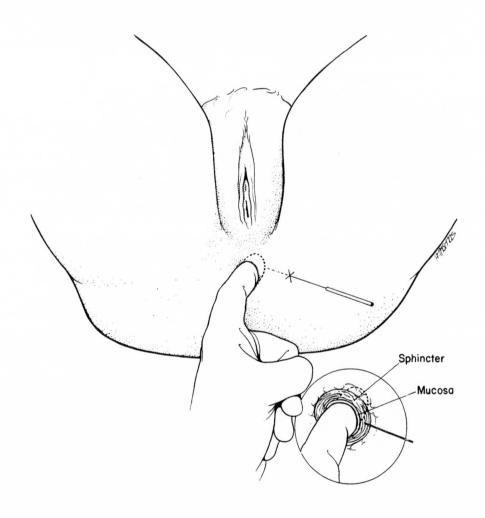

Innervation:

By the pudendal nerve (from S2–3–4 roots and anterior division of the sacral plexus).

Origin & Insertion:

This is a funnel shaped sphincter which is formed by the lowest most part of the levator ani muscle. Its fibers attach firmly to the coccyx in the back and the perineal body in the front.

Position:

The patient is in supine position with both legs in stirrups (GYN position) in order to expose widely the perineal region.

Electrode Insertion:

Bimanual maneuver is recommended. With the free hand gloved, the index finger is placed inside the anus with the pulp side of the finger "looking" to the hemisphincter under study. A 50mm electrode is inserted about two-fingers' breadth from the edge of the rectum. The finger placed inside the anus will guide the electrode to reach the proper placement and to prevent the tip from piercing the rectal mucosa. During this maneuver great care should be taken to avoid puncturing the examiner's finger with the electrode.

Test Maneuver:

The patient is asked to contract the sphincter as if trying to avoid having a bowel movement.

Pitfalls:

1) If too deep, it may penetrate the rectum space.
2) If too superficial, it will be in the gluteus maximus.

Comments:

1) The muscle is involved in unilateral or bilateral lesions of the pudendal nerve, at the pelvic level or at the sacral plexus, cauda equina or conus medullaris level.
2) This muscle is used as pick-up for the electrical evaluation of the

pudendal reflex (both hemisphincters should be tested for comparison reasons).

3) The natural tone of the sphincter keeps the canal and the anus closed; this closure can be tightened voluntarily by the patient.

B. SPHINCTER URETHRAE (URINARY SPHINCTER)

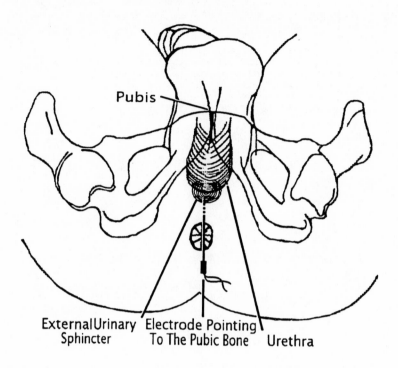

Pubis

ExternalUrinary   Electrode Pointing
   Sphincter   To The Pubic Bone   Urethra

Innervation:

By the pudendal nerve, from S2–3–4 roots and anterior division of the sacral plexus.

Origin & Insertion:

This muscle lies deep to the perineal membrane, forming a complete cuff of the urethra, just distal to the prostate. Peripheral fibers anchor to the perineal membrane, the inferior pubic rami and the perineal body.

Position:

The patient is in supine position with both legs in stirrups (GYN position) in order to expose the perineal region.

Electrode Insertion:

Bimanual maneuver is recommended. With the free hand gloved, the index finger is placed inside the rectum with the pulp side of the finger facing up. A 50mm or 75mm electrode is inserted two fingers breadth volar to the anus and through the perineal body. The electrode is directed upward and cephalad at an angle of about 45 toward the pubic bone. The finger placed within the rectum has to identify the lower pole of the prostate, and guide the electrode to enter the sphincter muscle which is located just distal to the prostate. During this maneuver great care should be taken in order to avoid puncturing the examiner's finger with the electrode.

Test Maneuver:

The patient is asked to contract the sphincter as if trying to avoid passing urine.

Pitfalls:

(1) If the electrode is directed
  (a) too volarly, it may enter the corpus spongiosum or the bulbo-spongiosus muscle.
  (b) Too dorsally, it will be in the rectal sphincter or enter the rectum.
  (c) Too deep, it will enter the prostate.

Comments:

(1) In females, the muscle is poorly developed and therefore it is very difficult to identify. On the other hand, the approach to this muscle is intravaginally which carries a significant risk of infection.
(2) This muscle is affected in unilateral or bilateral lesions of the pudendal nerve, sacral plexus, cauda equina, or conus medullaris. Paralysis of this muscle may result in urinary incontinence.

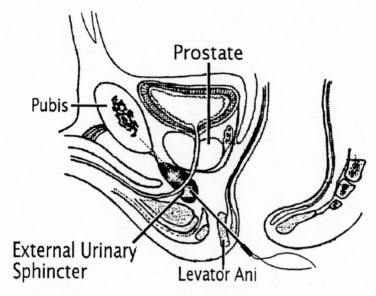

Figure 93. Cross section of the pelvic area showing the proper electrode insertion.

TRANSVERSUS PERINEAL SUPERFICIALIS

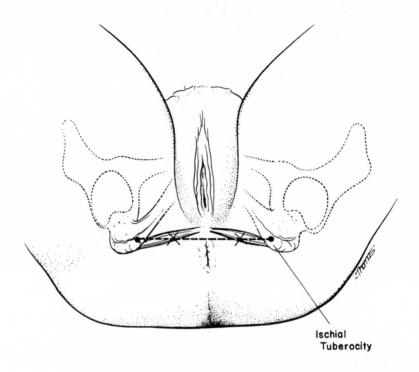

Ischial
Tuberocity

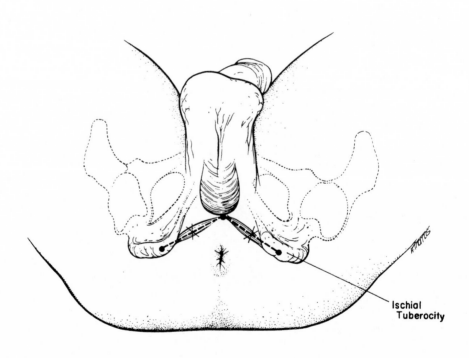

Ischial
Tuberocity

Innervation:

By perineal branch of pudendal nerve from S3–4 roots and anterior division of sacral plexus.

Origin:

From the ischial tuberosity following the posterior border of the perineal membrane.

Insertion:

Into the perineal body.

Position:

The patient is in supine position with both legs in stirrups (GYN position) in order to fully expose the perineal region.

Electrode Insertion:

In Female: The two ischial tuberosities are identified. An imaginary line joining them will pass between the posterior commissure of the vagina and the anus. The electrode is inserted on this line midway between the ischium and the perineal body. The length of the electrode will depend upon the thickness of the cellular layer. Usually a 50mm electrode is sufficient. *In Males:* The urethra is palpated in the ventral aspect of the shaft of the penis and followed posteriorly until it turns deep behind the pubis. At this point, an imaginary line is drawn to each ischial tuberosity. The electrode is inserted at the midpoint of this line.

Test Maneuver:

Its function is to fix the perineal body, therefore the patient is asked to contract the pelvic floor as if to prevent a bowel movement.

Pitfalls:

If the electrode is inserted too posteriorly, it will be in either the rectal sphincter or in the levator ani; too lateral, it will be in the ischiocavernosus; too anterior, it will be in the urethra (in males) or in the bulbo cavernosus (in females).

Comments:

1) This muscle, as all the other muscles in the perineal region that runs in a transverse direction helps support the prostate in males. In females it forms the limit between the urogenital diaphragm (anteriorly) and the anal triangle (posteriorly) and gives major support to these two structures.

2) This muscle is affected in lesions of the pudendal nerve, sacral plexus, cauda equina or conus medularis. In females, it can also be damaged as a result of delivering large babies (over stretching or rupture of the muscle). In multiparas, it may no longer have the strength nor sufficient tone to be a significant support for the pelvic viscerae.

SECTION XII
MUSCLES OF
THE PARASPINAL REGION

QUADRATUS LUMBORUM

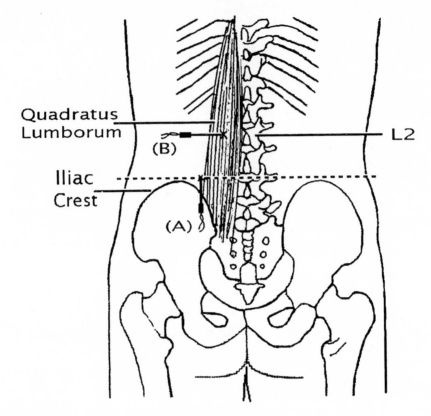

Innervation:

Ventral rami (from T12-L1-2-3)

Origin:

From the posterior two inches of the iliac crest and the iliolumbar ligament.

Insertion:

To lower border of last rib and transverse processes of upper 4 lumbar vertebrae.

Position:

The patient is in prone position.

Electrode Insertion:

The patient is asked to elevate the chest off the table to increase the lumbar lordosis, thus allowing the precise identification of the lateral border of the erector spinae muscle. Two areas can be chosen: (a) One-finger's breadth lateral to the erector spine mass and just proximal to the iliac crest: the electrode will travel through the latissimus dorsi aponeurosis before entering the quadratus lumborum. (b) The 2nd lumbar vertebra level is identified and the electrode is inserted three-fingers' breadth lateral to the spinous process. The electrode will travel through the latissimus dorsi aponeurosis and the erector spinae before entering the muscle. Because of the thickness and toughness of the lumbar aponeurosis, piercing it is easy to feel, which helps in appreciating where the tip of the electrode may be at any given time.

Test Maneuver:

The patient is asked to laterally bend the body, or to hike the hemipelvis on the ipsilateral side.

Pitfalls:

Approach (a): if the electrode is too superficial, it will be in the latissimus dorsi; if too medial, it will be in the erector spinae; if too lateral, it will be in the internal oblique. If too deep, it may enter the abdominal cavity.

Approach (b): if electrode is too superficial, it will be in the erector spinae; if too deep, it will be either in the psoas muscle (medially) or in the retroperitoneal renal space. If too medial, it will be in the multifidus; if too lateral, it will be in the renal space.

Comments:

This muscle is involved in lesions of the T12-L1 root, in A.H.C. diseases or degenerative conditions such as A.L.S. By attaching to the last rib, it extends the anchorage of the diaphragm to the iliac crest, therefore making it an important accessory respiratory muscle.

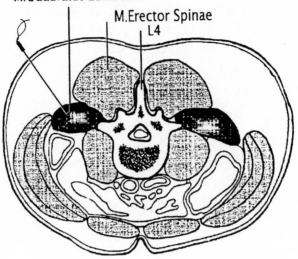

Figure 94. Cross section at the L4 level.

PARASPINALS

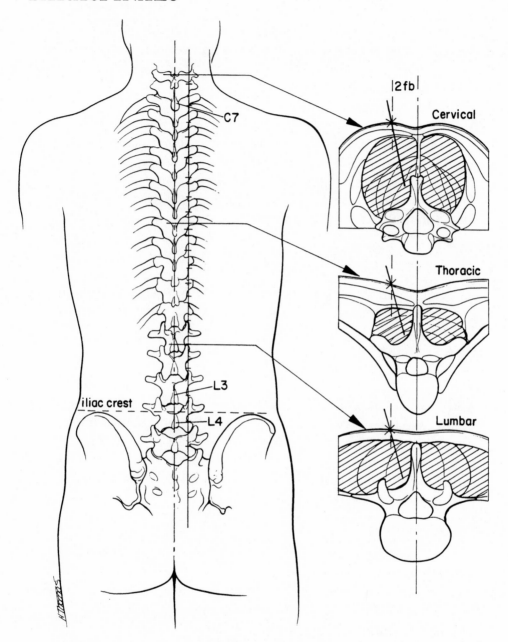

Paraspinal muscles are a generic anatomical term used to identify all those muscles located at each side of the spinous process of the spinal column. They are divided in 3 regions: the Cervical, the Thoracic, and the Lumbo-Sacral. All of these muscles are positioned in several layers and they are so close together that it is impossible to isolate them

277

individually for electrodiagnostic purposes. However, if the electrode is placed in the angle between the lamina of the vertebra and the spinous process, it will be in the multifidus.

Innervation:

All of these muscles are supplied by branches of the posterior division of the spinal nerve at their respective level. The innervation usually extends to one or two segments above and below a particular level. This creates a significant amount of overlapping innervation in the entire paraspinal groups. This anatomical characteristic makes it very difficult to assess the precise localization in cases of radicular compromise.

Origin and Insertion:

It is impossible to describe the origin and insertion of all paraspinals; this would be beyond the scope of this book. Suffice to say that the deeper the muscles, the shorter they are; the more superficial, the longer distance they travel.

Position:

The patient is in prone position. If the cervical area is to be studied, a pillow is placed across the chest of the patient, thus allowing the patient's head to flex and to rest on its forehead.
If the lumbo-sacral area is to be investigated, the pillow is placed across the abdomen, producing a mild "arching" of the lower spine. For the thoracic area, the patient is flat.

Electrode Insertion:

Prior to inserting the electrode, the level of the spine must be identified. Two landmarks are used: for the cervical and thoracic area, the spinous process of C7 (prominent) is identified and the count is done up or down accordingly. For the lumbo-sacral area, an imaginary line is drawn between the upper most part of the iliac crests. This line intersects the spinal column at the L3–L4 intervertebral level. The count proceeds up or down accordingly.
The electrode is inserted about one to two-finger breadths' from the spinous process of the identified level, down to the lamina of the vertebra.

Test Maneuver:

For the cervical area: The patient is asked to elevate or extend the head. If full relaxation cannot be obtained, the patient is asked to push the head onto the examining table.

For the lumbo-sacral area: The patient is asked to elevate the whole leg (from the hip) on the side under study.

If full relaxation cannot be obtained, the patient is asked to either push with the knee on the side under study onto the examining table, or slightly elevate the pelvis off the table.

Pitfalls:

If the electrode is too superficial, it may be in the superficial muscular layer of the back (trapezius; latissimus dorsi; rhomboids or splenius).

Comments:

The paraspinal muscles can be affected segmentally in processes involving the roots, the cauda equina, the conus medularis, vascular accidents involving the anterior spinal artery or in degenerative or inflammatory conditions involving the A.H.C. (polio, A.L.S.).

When studying the C7-T1 segment, care should be taken to avoid going too deep and accidentally causing damage to the sympathetic outflow, which results in unilateral Horner's syndrome (author experience).

SECTION XIII
MUSCLES OF
THE ABDOMINAL WALL

RECTUS ABDOMINAL

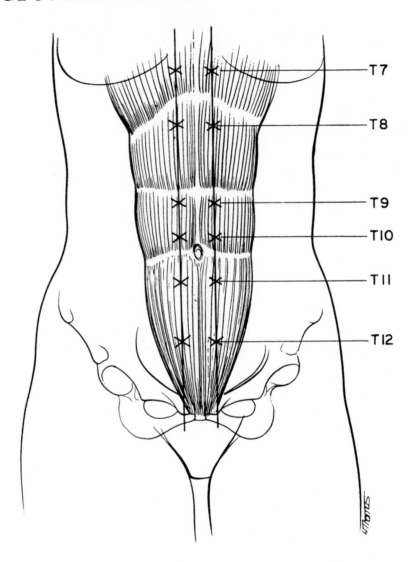

T7
T8
T9
T10
T11
T12

Innervation:

By intercostal T7–T12

Origin:

From the pubic crest and the ligament in front of the pubic symphysis. This muscle broadens as it travels upward at each side of the linea alba.

Insertion:

To the xiphoid process and over the costal margin to the 7th, 6th and 5th cartilages. In the supraumbilical portion this muscle is crossed by three horizontal tendinous intersections firmly attached to the anterior layer of the muscle aponeurotic sheath.

Position:

The patient is in supine position.

Electrode Insertion:

The electrode is inserted two-fingers' breadth lateral to the abdominal midline. The exact point of insertion will depend upon the intercostal nerve to be evaluated. The supraumbilical portion is supplied by T7-8-9; the umbilical portion by T10 and the infraumbilical portion by T11-T12.

Test Maneuver:

The patient is asked to lift the body off the table or if the patient cannot do it, to ask him to cough or to valsalva.

Pitfalls:

If the electrode is placed too lateral, it will be in the flat abdominal wall muscles. If it is too deep, it may enter the abdominal cavity.

Comments:

To prevent this accident from happening, one must pay attention to the piercing of the anterior aponeurosis. Once this is felt, the electrode is advanced very cautiously until a resistance is felt again. This represents the posterior aponeurosis and it *must not* be pierced.

In the upper most portion of the muscle, which rests over the rib cage, the insertion must be performed through the skin lying on top of a rib which will prevent further penetration. This muscle is affected in thoracic radiculopathies (very rare), in intercostal neuritis (herpetic); in anterior horn cell (A.H.C.) diseases (polio; amyotrophic lateral sclerosis (A.L.S.).

The paralysis or weakness of this muscle produces an obvious bulging of the anterior abdominal wall.

EXTERNAL OBLIQUE

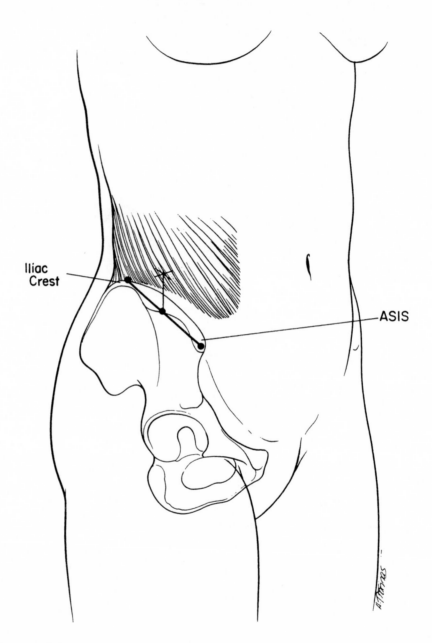

Innervation:

By the intercostal from T7–T12

Origin:

In the rib cage, from the 5th to the 12th ribs (interdigitate with the serratus anterior and latissimus dorsi). The posterior edge remains free and blends with the posterior lumbar fascia.

Insertion:

Into the outer lip of the anterior half of the iliac crest. The anterior edge of the muscle ends in a broad aponeurosis which runs anterior to the rectus abdominal muscle and joins the one from the opposite at the midline (linea alba).

Position:

The patient is in supine position.

Electrode Insertion:

The highest point in the iliac crest is identified as well as the anterior superior iliac spine (A.S.I.S.). Midway along this line, the electrode is inserted just cephalad to the iliac crest, until the aponeurosis is pierced.

Test Maneuver:

The patient is asked to lift the shoulder of the ipsilateral side off the table.

Pitfalls:

If the electrode is too deep (2nd aponeurosis is pierced), it will be in the internal oblique; if deeper yet (3rd aponeurosis is pierced), it will be in the transversus abdominal; if deeper yet, it will enter the abdominal cavity.

Comments:

This muscle is affected in thoracic radiculopathies (very rare) or intercostal neuritis (herpetic); in A.H.C. diseases (polio; A.L.S.). The paralysis or weakness of this muscle produces a flabby and protuberant lateral abdominal wall. The muscular fibers do not extend below the level of the A.S.I.C. nor medial to a vertical line drawn from the tip of the 9th costal cartilage.

SECTION XIV
INTERCOSTAL AND DIAPHRAGM MUSCLES

INTERCOSTALS

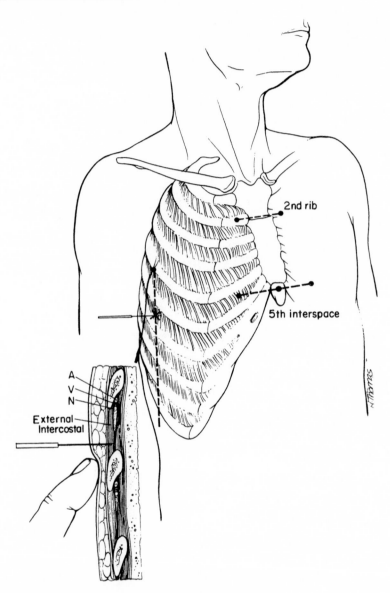

2nd rib

5th interspace

A
V
N
External
Intercostal

Innervation

Both, the internal and external intercostal by the anterior division of the spinal nerves from T1 to T11.

Origin

External: From the inferior border of the rib above.
Internal: From the floor of the costal groove above.

Insertion

Both muscles to the upper border of the rib below. The muscle fibers of the external intercostal are directed obliquely downwards and externally, while the fibers of the internal intercostal are directed also obliquely but 90 angle to the external (downward and vertebrally).

Position

The patient is in supine position.

Electrode Insertion

The most accessible area is the anterior axillary line. To count the ribs, two methods can be used: (1) identifying the angle of Lewis (junction between the manubrium and the body of the sternum). At each side of this angle the rib #2 inserts: counting downward, the intercostal space can be identified. (2) Identifying the xiphoid process, the 5th intercostal space can be identified at each side of it (between the 5th and 6th ribs). This space can be followed laterally toward the anterior axillary line, and the counting of the ribs can be done in an upward or downward direction. When the intended intercostal space is well identified, the free hand's index finger is positioned on the rib below and the electrode is then inserted just proximal to the finger and tangential to the upper edge of the rib. The progression of the electrode is stopped as soon as piercing the aponeurosis is felt. At this moment, electrical activity should be present with each inspiration.

Test Maneuver

The patient is asked to inspire.

Pitfalls

(1) If too deep, it may enter the pleural cavity with possible puncture of the lung underneath. If there is any doubt during the procedure, a chest X ray should be taken. I do not believe X ray should be a routine test in all patients.
(2) If the electrode is too superficial, it may be in any of the muscles that attach to the chest wall (latissimus dorsi; serratus anterior, pectoralis major; pectoralis minor) depending upon the intercostal muscle under investigation.

(3) If the electrode is placed too close to the lower edge of the proximal rib, the neurovascular bundle can be injured.

Comments

This muscle can be involved in thoracic radiculopathies (very rare); in
intercostal neuritis (herpetic); in A.H.C. diseases (polio; A.L.S.).
The intercostal muscles are inspiratory muscles. They contract only in
forced expiration.
The paralysis of these muscles produces a significant decrease in
amplitude of the rib cage in normal breathing.
In obese individuals or in females with large breasts, it could be
difficult to identify the appropriate intercostal space.

DIAPHRAGM

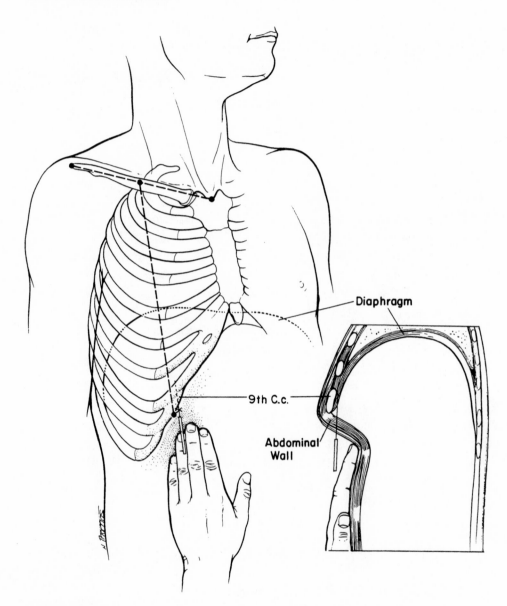

Diaphragm

9th C.c.

Abdominal Wall

Innervation

By phrenic nerves (C3-4-5) and peripherally by lower intercostal nerves (T6–11).

Origin

From the thoracic outlet (last 6 ribs): it is divided into several portions: sternal, costal, vertebrocostal and lumbar or vertebral part.

Insertion

To a strong central tendon that is pierced by the inferior vena cava.

Position

Patient in supine position.

Electrode Insertion

(1) The 9th rib cartilage is localized at the point where the paramedial-clavicular line intersects the rib cage. This line is identified by drawing a line from a point midway between the sternal notch and the lateral end of the clavicle (medial to the midclavicular line). The intersection of this line with the margin of the rib cage corresponds approximately to the angle formed by the rib cage and the rectus abdominus muscle. A 50mm monopolar electrode is used. With his free hand, the electromyographer firmly and continuously depresses the abdominal wall just distal to the rib cage. In this way the costal margin is sharply delineated. The electrode is inserted in a direction parallel to the posterior aspect of the chest wall. The electrode will travel through the skin, subcutaneous tissue, and abdominal wall muscles (these muscles will show electrical activity if the patient is not relaxed). By continuing to advance the electrode, it will enter the costal insertion of the diaphragm.*

Test Maneuver

The regular patient's breathing will produce bursts of electrical activity during inspiration which will alternate with electrical silence during expiration. A deep inspiration will produce a sustained activity which will last the whole length of the inspiration effort.

Pitfalls

(1) If electrode is introduced perpendicular to the skin without a sharp delineation of the costal margin, it may penetrate the abdominal cavity.
(2) If electrode remains too superficial, it will be in the abdominal wall muscles.

---

*P.B. Saadeh, C.F. Crisafulli, J. **Sosner,** and E. **Wolf,** Needle electromyography of the diaphragm: A new technique, *Muscle and Nerve,* 16: 15–20, 1993.

(3) If the electrode is inserted more than 4–5 cm in depth, it may reach the pleural cavity.

Comments

(1) The diaphragm presents three large openings: (a) vena cava (tendon portion) at the lower 8th thoracic vertebra level, (b) esophageal opening (through the right crus at the 10th thoracic vertebra level, (c) aortic opening in front of the 12th thoracic vertebra.

(2) The lesion of the phrenic nerve can occur at the neck and at the mediastinum (commonly by tumors or adenopathies) or in high spinal cord injuries. In the former conditions the respiration of the patient may not be affected (especially if it is unilateral). In the latter, the respiration is severely affected and the patient may die if proper respiratory support is not administered rapidly.

(3) In cervical spinal cord lesions at or distal to C5, the function of this muscle will be enough to keep the patient alive.

(4) Although the phrenic nerve is mainly a motor nerve, one-third of its fibers are sensory and they supply the pleura and pericardium.

(5) Irritation of this nerve is common and causes an attack of hiccups.

(6) In obese people, it may be very difficult to identify the proper landmarks; trying in these people may become dangerous. If in doubt, the investigation should be cancelled.

APPENDIX

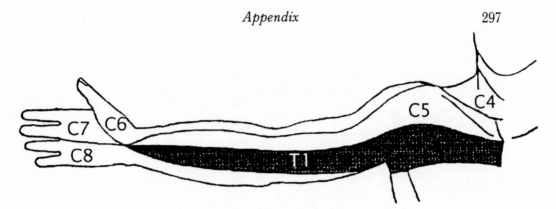

Figure 95. Dermatomal distribution of the anterior aspect of the upper extremity.

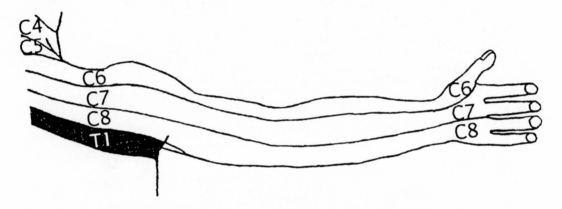

Figure 96. Dermatomal distribution of the posterior aspect of the upper extremity.

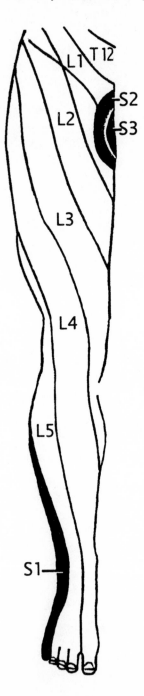

Figure 97. Dermatomal distribution of the anterior aspect of the lower extremity.

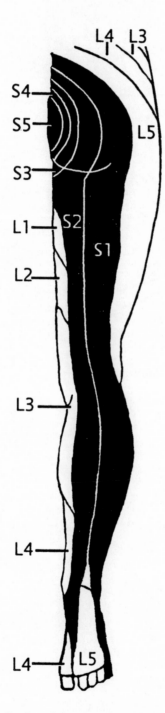

Figure 98. Dermatomal distribution of the posterior aspect of the leg and gluteal region.

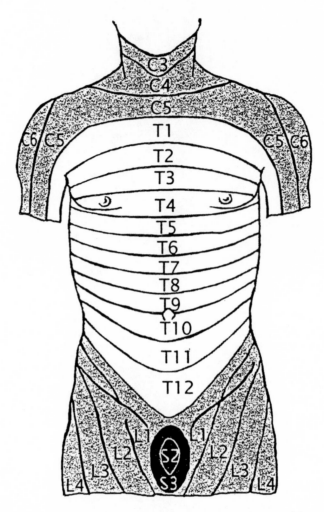

Figure 99. Dermatomal distribution of the anterior aspect of the trunk.

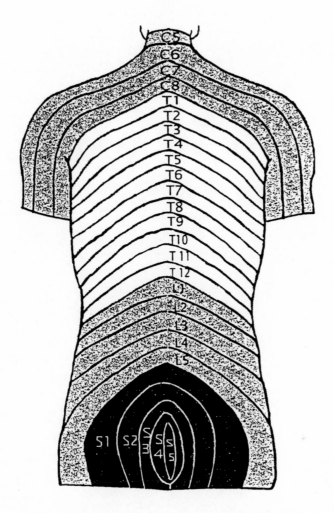

Figure 100. Dermatomal distribution of the posterior aspect of the trunk.

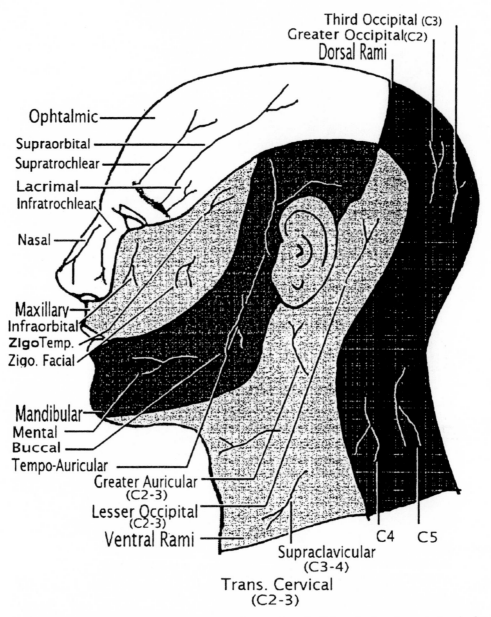

Figure 101. Dermatomal distribution of the face and neck. Trigeminal and cervical spinal nerves coverage.

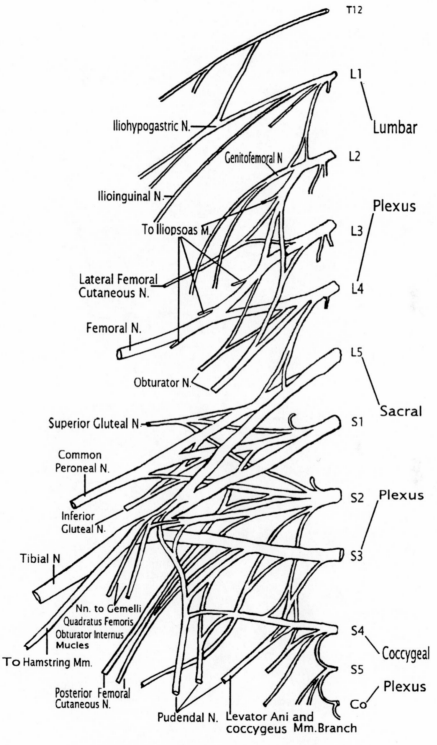

Figure 102. The lumbo-sacral-coccygeal plexus.

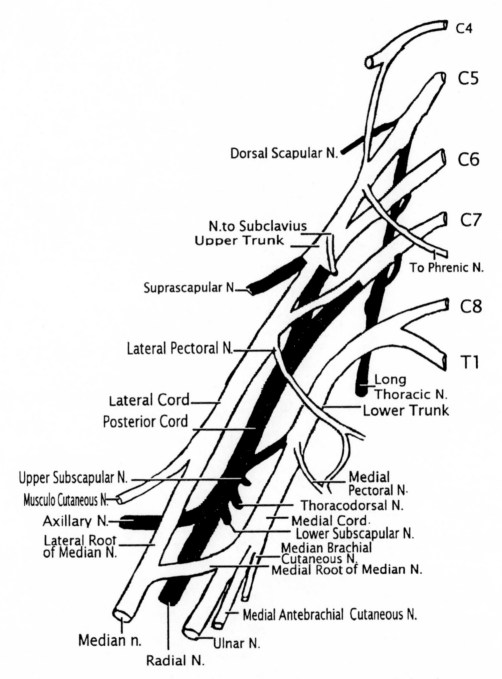

Figure 103. The brachial plexus; posterior components were darkened.

MUSCLE INNERVATION FOR ALL MUSCLES SHOWN IN THIS BOOK

	peripheral nerve	brachial plexus			
		cord	division	trunk	root
abductor digiti minimi	ulnar	medial	anterior	lower	C8-T1
abductor pollicis brevis	median	medial	anterior	lower	C8-T1
adductor pollicis	ulnar	medial	anterior	lower	C8-T1
dorsal interosseous	ulnar	medial	anterior	lower	C8-T1
volar interosseious	ulnar	medial	anterior	lower	C8-T1
lumbricals (1–2)	median	medial	anterior	lower	C8-T1
lumbricals (3–4)	ulnar	medial	anterior	lower	C8-T1
flexor pollicis brevis (sup. head)	median	medial	anterior	lower	C8-T1
flexor pollicis brevis (deep head)	ulnar	medial	anterior	lower	C8-T1
opponens digiti minimi	ulnar	medial	anterior	lower	C8-T1
opponens pollicis	median	medial	anterior	lower	C8-T1
abductor pollicis longus	post interos. (radial)	posterior	posterior	middle & lower	C7-C8
anconeus	radial	posterior	posterior	middle & lower	C7-C8
brachioradialis	radial	posterior	posterior	upper	C5-C6
extensor carpi radialis (longus & brevis)	radial	posterior	posterior	upper & middle	C6-C7
extensor carpa ulnaris	post interos. (radial)	posterior	posterior	upper, middle & lower	C6-C7-C8
extensor digitor comminus extensor digiti minimi proprius	post interos. (radial)	posterior	posterior	middle & lower	C7-C8
extensor indici proprius	post interos. (radial)	posterior	posterior	middle & lower	C7-C8
extensor pollicis brevis	post interos. (radial)	posterior	posterior	middle & lower	C7-C8
extensor pollicis congus	post interos. (radial)	posterior	posterior	middle & lower	C7-C8
flexor carpi radialis	median	lateral & medial	anterior	upper, middle & lower	C6-C7-C8
flexor carpi ulnaris	ulnar	medial	anterior	lower	C8-T1
flexor digitorum profundus (#2–3)	ant. interos. (median)	medial	anterior	middle & lower	C7-C8

	peripheral nerve	brachial plexus			
		cord	division	trunk	root
flexor digitorum profundus (#4–5)	ulnar	medial	anterior	lower	C8-T1
flexor digitorum sublimis	median	lateral medial	anterior	middle lower	C7-C8-T1
flexor pollicis longus	ant. interos. (median)	lateral medial	anterior	middle lower	C7-C8-T1
palmaris longus	median	lateral medial	anterior	middle lower	C7-C8-T1
pronator quadratus	ant. interos. (median)	lateral medial	anterior	middle lower	C7-C8-T1
pronator teres	median	lateral	anterior	upper & middle	C6-C7
supinator	post interos. (radial)	posterior	posterior	upper	C5-C6
biceps brachii	musculo-cutaneous	lateral	anterior	upper	C5-C6
brachialis	musculo-cutaneous	lateral	anterior	upper	C5-C6
coraco-brachialis	musculo-cutaneous	lateral	anterior	upper & middle	C6-C7
triceps	radial	posterior	posterior	middle & lower	C7-C8-T1
deltoid	axillary	posterior	posterior	upper	C5-C6
infraspinatus	suprascapular	—	—	upper	C5-C6
latissimus dorsi	thoraco dorsal	posterior	posterior	upper, middle & lower	C6-C7-C8
pectoralis major (clavicular)	lateral pectoral	lateral	anterior	upper	C5-C6
pectoralis major (sterno-costal)	medial pectoral	medial	anterior	middle & lower	C7-C8-T1
supraspinatus	suprascapular			upper	C5-C6
teres major	lower scapular	posterior	posterior	upper	C5-C6
teres minor	axillary	posterior	posterior	upper	C5-C6
levator scapulae	dorsal scapular twigs from				C5 C3-C4
pectoralis minor	medial & lateral pectoral	medial & lateral	anterior	upper, middle & lower	C6-C7-C8

	peripheral nerve		*brachial plexus*		
		cord	division	trunk	root
rhomboideus major	dorsal scapular				C5
rhomboideus minor	dorsal scapular				C5
serratus anterior	long thoracic				C5-C6-C7
trepezius	accessory (c.n. #11) (spinal portion) nerve twigs from				C3-C4

	peripheral nerve			*L-S plexus* division	root
abductor digiti quinti	lateral plantar	tibial	sciatic	ventral	S1-S2
abductor hallucis	medial plantar	tibial	sciatic	ventral	S1-S2
adductor hallucis	lateral plantar	tibial	sciatic	ventral	S1-S2
extensor digitorum brevis	deep peroneal	common peroneal	sciatic	dorsal	L5-S1
flexor digitorum brevis	medial plantar	tibial	sciatic	ventral	S1-S2
flexor digiti quinti	lateral plantar	tibial	sciatic	ventral	S1-S2
flexor hallucis brevis	medial plantar	tibial	sciatic	ventral	S1-S2
interossei	lateral plantar	tibial	sciatic	ventral	S1-S2
quadratus plantae	lateral plantar	tibial	sciatic	ventral	S1-S2
extensor digitorum longus	deep peroneal	common peroneal	sciatic	posterior	L5-S1
extensor hallucis longus	deep peroneal	common peroneal	sciatic	posterior	L5-S1
flexor digitorum longus		tibial	sciatic	ventral	L5-S1-S2
flexor hallicis longus gastrocnemius (lat. & median heads)		tibial	sciatic	ventral	L5-S1-S2
		tibial	sciatic	ventral	S1-S2
peroneus brevis	Superficial peroneal	common peroneal	sciatic	posterior	L5-S1-S2
peroneus longus	Superficial peroneal	common peroneal	sciatic	posterior	L5-S1-S2
peroneus tertius	deep peroneal	common peroneal	sciatic	posterior	L5-S1

	peripheral nerve			L-S plexus division	root
popliteus		tibial	sciatic	anterior	L5-S1
soleus		tibial	sciatic	anterior	L5-S1-S2
tibialis anterior	deep peroneal	common peroneal	sciatic	posterior	L4-L5
tibialis posterior		tibial	sciatic	anterior	L5-S1
adductor brevis	obturator nerve			anterior	L2-L3-L4
adductor longus	obturator nerve			anterior	L2-L3-L4
adductor magnus	obturator nerve			anterior	L2-L3- L4-L5
biceps femoris (long head)			sciatic (tibial portion)	anterior	L5-S1
biceps femoris (short head)			sciatic (peroneal port.)	posterior	L5-S1-S2
gracilis	obturator			anterior	L2-L3-L4
iliopsoas	femoral			posterior	L2-L3-L4
pectineus	femoral			posterior	L2-L3-L4
rectus femoris	femoral			posterior	L2-L3-L4
sartorius	femoral			posterior	L2-L3-L4
semimembranosus			sciatic (tibial port.)	anterior	L5-S1-S2
semitenoinosus			sciatic (tibial port.)	anterior	L5-S1-S2
tenso fascie latae	superior gluteal			posterior	L5-S1-S2
vastus intermedius	femoral			posterior	L2-L3-L4
vastus lateralis	femoral			posterior	L2-L3-L4
vastus medialis	femoral			posterior	L2-L3-L4
gluteus maximus	inferior gluteal nerve			posterior division	 L5-S1-S2

	peripheral nerve		*L-S plexus division*	*root*
gluteus medius	superior gluteal nerve		posterior division	L4-L5-S1
gluteus minimum	superior gluteal nerve		posterior division	L4-L5-S1
obturator internus and gemelci	obturaton internus nerve		anterior division	L5-S1-S2
piriformis	piriformis nerve			S1-S2
quadratus femoris	quadratus femoris nerve	sciatic (tibial portion)	anterior division	L4-S1-S2

	peripheral nerve	*branch*
retro auricular	facial (C.N. #7)	postauricular
orbicularis oculi	facial (C.N. #7)	temporal
dilator naris	facial (C.N. #7)	deep buccal
orbicularis oris	facial (C.N. #7)	superficial buccal
occipital frontalis	facial (C.N. #7)	temporal
tongue	hypoglossal (C.N. #12)	
sterno-cleido-mastoid	spinal accessory (C.N. #11)	spinal portion twigs from C3-C4
trapezius	spinal accessory (C.N. #11)	spinal portion twigs from C3-C4
temporal	trigeminal (C.N. #5)	deep temporal } from the
masseter	trigeminal (C.N. #5)	masseter } mandibular nerve
cricothyroid	vagus (C.N. #10)	superior laryngeal
thyroarytenoid	vagus (C.N. #10)	recurrent laryngeal
rectal sphincter	pudendal	anterior division sacral plexus
urinary sphincter	pudendal	anterior division sacral plexus
transverse perineal superficialis	pudendal	anterior division sacral plexus
quadratus lumborum	spinal	ventral division T12-L3
paraspinals	spinal	dorsal division
rectus abdominal	intercostals	T7-T12
external oblique	intercostals	T7-T12
intercostals	spinal	ventral division T1-T11
diaphragm	phenic	(C3-4-5)
	lower intercostals	(T6-11)